WOMEN AT HIGH RISK TO BREAST CANCER

DEVELOPMENTS IN ONCOLOGY

Recent volumes

M.J. van Zwieten, The rat as Animal Model in Breast Cancer: A Histopathological Study of Radiation- and Hormone-Induced Rat Mammary Tumors. ISBN 0-89838-624-1
B. Löwenberg and A. Hagenbeek, eds., Minimal Residual Disease in Acute Leukemia. ISBN 0-89838-630-6
I. van der Waal and G.B. Snow, eds., Oral Oncology. ISBN 0-89838-631-4
B.W. Hancock and A.H. Ward, eds., Immunological Aspects of Cancer. ISBN 0-89838-664-0
K.V. Honn and B.F. Sloan, Hemostatic Mechanisms and Metastasis. ISBN 0-89838-667-5
K.R. Harrap, W. Davis and A.H. Calvert, eds., Cancer Chemotherapy and Selective Drug Development. ISBN 0-89838-673-X
C.J.H. van de Velde and P.H. Sugarbaker, eds., Liver Metastasis. ISBN 0-89838-648-5
D.J. Ruiter, K. Welvaart and S. Ferrone, eds., Cutaneous Melanoma and Precursor Lesions. ISBN 0-89838-689-6
S.B. Howelll, ed., Intra-arterial and Intracavitary Cancer Chemotherapy. ISBN 0-89838-691-8
D.L. Kisner and J.F. Smyth, eds., Interferon Alpha-2: Pre-Clinical and Clinical Evaluation. ISBN 0-89838-701-9
P. Furmanski, J.C. Hager and M.A. Rich, eds., RNA Tumor Viruses, Oncogenes, Human Cancer and AIDs: On the Frontiers of Understanding. ISBN 0-89838-703-5
J. Talmadge, I.J. Fidler and R.. Oldham, Screening for Biological Response Modifiers: Methods and Rationale. ISBN 0-89838-712-4
J.C. Bottino, R.W. Opfell and F.M. Muggia, eds., Liver Cancer. ISBN 0-89838-713-2
P.K. Pattengale, R.J. Lukes and C.R. Taylor, Lymphoproliferative Diseases: Pathogenesis, Diagnosis Therapy. ISBN 0-89838-725-6
F. Cavalli, G. Bonadonna and M. Rozencweig, eds., Malignant Lymphomasa nd Hodgkin's Disease: Experimental and Therapeutic Advances. ISBN 0-89838-727-2
L. Baker, F. Valeriote and V. Ratanatharathorn, eds., Biology and Therapy of Acute Leukemia. ISBN 0-89838-728-0
J. Russo, ed., Immunocytochemistry in Tumor Diagnosis. ISBN 0-89838-737-X
R.L. Ceriani, ed., Monoclonal Antibodies and Breast Cancer. ISBN 0-89838-739-6
D.E. Peterson, G.E. Elias and S.T. Sonis, eds., Head and Neck Management of the Cancer Patient. ISBN 0-89838-747-7
D.M. Green, Diagnosis and Management of Malignant Solid Tumors in Infants and Children ISBN 0-89838-750-7
K.A. Foon and A.C. Morgan, Jr., eds., Monoclonal Antibody Therapy of Human Cancer. ISBN 0-89838-754-X
J.G. McVie, W. Bakker, Sj.Sc. Wagenaar and D. Carney, eds., Clinical and Experimental Pathology of Lung Cancer. ISBN 0-89838-764-7
K.V. Honn, W.E. Powers and B.F. Sloan, eds., Mechanisms of Cancer Metastasis. ISBN 0-89838-765-5
K. Lapis, L.A. Liotta and A.S. Rabson, eds., Biochemistry and Molecular Genetics of Cancer Metastasis. 0-89838-785-X
A.J. Mastromarino, ed., Biology and Treatment of Colorectal Metastasis. ISBN 0-89838-786-8
M.A. Rich, J.C. Hager and J. Taylor-Papadimitriou, eds., Breast Cancer: Origins, Detection and Treatment. ISBN 0-89838-792-2
D.G. Poplack, L. Massimo and P. Cornaglia-Ferraris, eds., The Role of Pharmacology in Pediatric Oncology. ISBN 0-89838-795-7
A. Hagenbeek and B. Löwenberg, eds., Minimal Residual Disease in Acute Leukemia 1986. ISBN 0-89838-799-X
F.M. Muggia and M. Rozencweig, eds., Clinical Evaluations of Antitumor Therapy. ISBN 0-89838-803-1
F.A. Valeriote and L. Baker, eds., Biochemical Modulation of Anticancer Agents: Experimental and Clinical Approaches. ISBN 0-89838-827-9
B.A. Stoll, ed., Pointers to Cancer Prognosis. ISBN 0-89838-841-4
K.H. Hollmann and J.M. Verley, eds., New Frontiers in Mammary Pathology 1986. ISBN 089838-852-X
D.J. Ruiter, G.J. Fleuren and S.O. Warnaar, eds., Application of Monoclonal Antibodies in Tumor Pathology. ISBN 0-89838-853-8
M. Chatel, F. Darcel and J. Pecker, eds., Brain Oncology. ISBN 0-89838-954-2
J.R. Ryan and L.O. Baker, eds., Recent Concepts in Sarcoma Treatment. ISBN 0-89838-376-5
M.A. Rich, J.C. Hager and D.M. Lopez, eds., Breast Cancer: Scientific and Clinical Aspects. ISBN 0-89838-387-0

WOMEN AT HIGH RISK TO BREAST CANCER

edited by

BASIL A. STOLL
Honorary Consultant Physician to Oncology Department,
St. Thomas' Hospital and to Joint Breast Clinic,
Royal Free Hospital, London, UK

KLUWER ACADEMIC PUBLISHERS
DORDRECHT / BOSTON / LONDON

Published by Kluwer Academic Publishers,
PO Box 17, 3300 AA Dordrecht, The Netherlands.

Kluwer Academic Publishers incorporates
the publishing programmes of
D. Reidel, Martinus Nijhoff, Dr W. Junk and MTP Press.

Sold and distributed in the USA and Canada
by Kluwer Academic Publishers,
101 Philip Drive, Norwell, MA 02061, USA.

In all other countries, sold and distributed
by Kluwer Academic Publishers Group,
PO Box 322, 3300 AH Dordrecht, The Netherlands.

Library of Congress Cataloging-in-Publication Data

Women at high risk to breast cancer.

(Developments in oncology)
Includes index.
1. Breast – Cancer – Etiology. 2. Breast – Cancer – Prevention. 3. Breast – Cancer – Epidemiology.
I. Stoll, Basil A. (Basil Arnold) II. Series.
[DNLM: 1. Breast Neoplasms – familial & genetic.
2. Breast Neoplasms – prevention & control. 3. Risk.
W1 DE998N / WP 870 W872]
RC280.B8W66 1988 616.99'449071 88-26610
ISBN 0-89838-416-8

Printed in Great Britain by Butler & Tanner Limited, Frome and London

Contents

Preface

Breast cancer is on the increase throughout the Western world where it is a major source of anxiety among women. The disease is also becoming more frequent in Asian and South American countries where once it was relatively uncommon. Multiple factors are suspected of promoting the disease and the increasing risk is attributed to recent changes in life-style and diet. This book is intended to provide an authoritative and balanced survey of the latest research into the genetic, familial, hormonal, reproductive, nutritional, social and geographic factors known to be associated with an increased predisposition to the disease.

Because of the overwhelming evidence that breast cancer has already disseminated by the time the tumour is large enough to be felt, there is increasing pressure for earlier diagnosis. There are reports that well organised mass screening programmes can lead to improved survival rates and there are pressures for population screening. If such programmes are to be pursued they must be highly efficient, and associated with intensive health education if they are to avoid creating undue anxiety among women who are invited to participate.

Although all women are potentially at risk for breast cancer, we need to develop a risk index to recognise women with a high degree of risk who need intensive monitoring. Such women will require skilful counselling. Although recent research suggests that hormonal manipulation or dietary change may delay progression of the disease to the malignant phase, careful planning is required if women are to be directed into suitable clinical trials of preventive methods.

This book should be useful not only for clinicians and epidemiologists but also for health educators, counsellors, nurses and psychosocial professionals. Being interdisciplinary, it has been written with a fully practical approach and quotes only the most recent and seminal references. I must express my thanks to the contributors who rose to this challenge. In order to make each chapter complete in itself, it was found necessary to permit a small degree of overlap with others.

BASIL A. STOLL
London
1989

List of Contributors

Joern Beckman, PhD
Assistant Professor, Department of Psychology, Universities of Odense and Aarhus; Chief Psychologist, Odense University Hospital, Denmark

William D. Dupont, PhD
Associate Professor of Biostatistics, Department of Preventive Medicine, Vanderbilt University School of Medicine, Nashville, Tennessee, USA

Ruth Ellman, MRCP, MFCM
Deputy Director, DHSS Screening Evaluation Unit; Senior Lecturer in Epidemiology, Institute of Cancer Research, London, UK

M. Jawed Iqbal, PhD
Senior Lecturer, Tumour Biology Unit, Rayne Institute, King's College School of Medicine, London, UK

Stephanie J. London, MD
Department of Epidemiology, Harvard School of Public Health, Boston, Massachusetts, USA

Henry T. Lynch, MD
Professor and Chairman, Department of Preventive Medicine and Public Health, Creighton University School of Medicine and The Hereditary Cancer Consultation Center, Omaha, Nebraska, USA

Jane F. Lynch, BSN
Department of Preventive Medicine and Public Health, Creighton University School of Medicine and The Hereditary Cancer Consultation Center, Omaha, Nebraska, USA

Joseph N. Marcus, MD
Department of Pathology, Creighton University School of Medicine and The Hereditary Cancer Consultation Center, Omaha, Nebraska, USA

Curtis Mettlin, PhD
Director, Cancer Control and Epidemiology, Roswell Park Memorial Institute, Buffalo, New York, USA

A.B. Miller, MB, FRCP(C), FRCP
Professor, Department of Preventive Medicine and Biostatistics; Director, National Breast Screening Study, Faculty of Medicine, University of British Columbia, Vancouver, BC, Canada

David L. Page, MD
Professor of Pathology and Associate Professor of Epidemiology, Vanderbilt University School of Medicine, Nashville, Tennessee, USA

M.T. Schechter, MD, MSc, PhD
Assistant Professor and National Health Scholar, Department of Health Care and Epidemiology, Faculty of Medicine, University of British Columbia, Vancouver, BC, Canada

Elinor R. Schoenfeld, PhD
Department of Cancer Control and Epidemiology, Roswell Park Memorial Institute, Buffalo, New York, USA

Basil A. Stoll, FRCR, FFR
Consulting Physician, Department of Oncology, St. Thomas' Hospital, and to Joint Breast Clinic, Royal Free Hospital, London, UK

W. Taylor, PhD, MIBiol
Reader in Steroid Biochemistry, Department of Physiological Sciences, The Medical School, University of Newcastle upon Tyne, UK

Patrice Watson, PhD
Department of Preventive Medicine and Public Health, Creighton University School of Medicine and The Hereditary Cancer Consultation Center, Omaha, Nebraska, USA.

Walter C. Willett, MD, Dr.PH
Professor of Nutritional Epidemiology, Harvard School of Public Health, Boston, Massachusetts, USA

PART ONE

WHO IS AT HIGH RISK?

Chapter 1

In Search of Guidelines

BASIL A. STOLL

The expectations of the 1950s have not been fulfilled and the number of women dying from breast cancer has increased over the past 30 years both in the UK and the USA [1, 2]. It appears that earlier diagnosis and claims of more effective treatments have not been reflected by improvement in the 5 year survival rates of treated cases over the past 15 years [3]. How then are we going to reduce deaths from breast cancer in the Western world? While we may develop more effective agents for eradicating the tumour once it has disseminated, an alternative is to develop more effective methods of detecting the primary tumour before it has disseminated or, better still, of arresting it at an even earlier stage.

This book is concerned with the latter goals. It examines the current guidelines on: (a) how to recognise those individuals who are most at risk to the development of breast cancer; (b) how to screen and monitor these women in order to detect the earliest evidence of cancer; and (c) how the progression of the primary lesion may be arrested in an attempt to prevent the cancer from manifesting clinically. The following chapters set out the current guidelines for each procedure against the background of the latest scientific evidence.

But to select a monitoring or protection programme for a women who is thought to be at high risk to breast cancer involves more than a consideration of guidelines. Because of the uncertainties, choices must involve value judgements both by the women and by the physician. For each individual women, the possible benefit must be weighed against the trouble, expense and anxiety attached to the procedure, and if the facilities are provided by the state, they must be proved worthwhile [4]. This chapter provides an introductory perspective and also examines the cost-benefit ratio of monitoring and protection programmes, not only from the point of view of the individual but also that of society in general.

Guidelines for Assessing Individual Risk

Most cancers result from the interaction of genetic and environmental factors in the individual. The popular media give the impression that most cancer are preventable or, failing that, would be cured if only they were caught in time. Yet, despite impressive advance in medical research the overall mortality rate in the West from all types of cancer is not falling [1, 2]. One major reason is that in the Western world, people are living longer, and because the risk for most cancers increases progressively with age, men and women are increasingly likely to manifest one cancer or another before they die. For example, elderly men dying of other causes frequently show undiagnosed small, slowly growing cancers in the prostate, while similar occult cancers in the breast are found in many elderly women.

However, deaths from breast cancer among young and middle-aged women are also increasing and this suggests other possible causes for the increased numbers of breast cancer. Prominent are the marked changes which have occurred in the patterns of diet, childbearing and breast feeding in Western society in the past two generations. These provide 'risk factors' which have been shown to increase a woman's susceptibility to breast cancer. Thus, until we can recognise biological markers of susceptibility (such as chromosomal abnormality or evidence of past virus infection in breast tissue) we can rely only on clinical markers such as a family history of breast cancer or specific characteristics in a women's reproductive history or life style. These clinical risk factors are used also to select women who require active intervention, whether by regular monitoring or by some attempt at protection.

The problem is that the group identified in this way may not be at very high risk, or else that the group may be so large that it does not effectively limit the numbers to be kept under surveillance. Because there are several clinical risk factors for breast cancer, about 95% of women have at least one of them. For practical purposes, it is also important that such risk factors should be easy to recognise, reliable and reasonably common, because even if strongly predictive yet rare, surveillance of such women will not make much impact on the overall problem.

Thus, in order to decide how surveillance should be practised, we need first to assess which of the suspected risk factors are most useful and then how to combine them to identify women at *very high* risk. It might also be useful to identify those at *very low* risk to breast cancer, because surveillance might be relaxed in such women. However, it would be dangerous to restrict screening only to those with high risk criteria because women with low risk criteria still have about four fifths the risk of the average women of developing breast cancer (see Chapter 7). It is claimed that by excluding low risk women from screening, we might eliminate the possibility of early detection of two thirds of all new cases of breast cancer [5].

How do we quantitate the degree of increased risk which a women may have of developing breast cancer? Relatively few women may be said to be at the highest risk if we define that as about four times as great as that in the general population. However, some measurement of a woman's risk is needed to make the difficult choice between regular monitoring and some advice on protection. For example, in a women with two risk factors, one might advise shorter intervals between screening examinations, while in a women with three or more major risk factors one might consider offering her participation in a clinical trial of a 'cancer prevention' regime (see Chapter 10).

In addition, in order to distinguish those women who need only regular monitoring from those from whom advice on protection is justified, we need to establish the relative strength of each known risk factor – whether it is strongly or weakly predictive. We also need to establish the independence of one risk factor from another because adding together two risk factors which are interrelated may give a false impression of higher risk. For example, it is well established that women who have attended university have a relatively higher predisposition to breast cancer, but such women are also more likely to have delayed their first pregnancy, and this is clearly the real risk factor.

Of the factors thought to determine a woman's likelihood of manifesting breast cancer, the strongest are advancing age, residence in a Western country and a history of breast cancer in a mother or sister appearing before the menopause. Of relatively less importance are a family history of the disease appearing after the menopause, delay before having the first baby, a record of early onset of menstruation or of delayed onset of the menopause or a record of a breast biopsy which showed evidence of atypia in the cells (see Chapter 5). Caucasian race, higher social class, obesity and incomplete breast feeding are additional risk factors. Evidence for the risk associated with each of these different factors is discussed in detail in later chapters.

Guidelines for Monitoring High Risk Families

The monitoring of women with a family history of breast cancer requires their education as to their degree of risk (see Chapter 3). Counselling of high risk families needs to be careful and thorough, and it is essential to stress to members of the family that the disease is not inherited [6]. Only the genes which make a women susceptible to the disease are inherited, and if the cancer is to proceed to the fully invasive stage, it requires a series of promoting steps involving a women's diet, life style and environmental factors. These are the factors which lie, at least in part, within a women's control.

There are now known to be over 200 hereditary chromosomal abnormalities which are associated with an increased susceptibility to cancer of one type or another [7]. However, individuals with these conditions account for only a small fraction of all human cancers. A hereditary basis for cancer susceptibility may involve an increased sensitivity of some cells to cancer-initiating factors such as natural radiation, viruses or chemicals. Alternatively, it may involve a natural deficiency of enzymes which normally dispose of cancer-inducing chemicals, whether derived from the environment or produced inside the body.

It is important that women should be informed that familial susceptibility to cancer is generally site-specific, meaning that a family history of different types of cancer at different sites of the body in various relatives is irrelevant except in rare cases (see Chapter 3). In the context of breast cancer risk, a history of the disease having occurred in one's mother in both breasts and before the menopause is however, a very high risk factor. (Familial cancers of all types tend to show multiple points of origin and tend also to manifest at a younger age group than would similar cancers occurring randomly.)

There are some rare families where males as well as females show an increased risk of breast cancer [8]. In general however, the vast majority of breast cancers occur randomly in women with no obvious family history of that type of cancer. They are presumed to result from damage to genes by chemicals, viruses or radiation such as is accumulated by every individual during the course of life. Some is repaired, some leads to death of the affected cell while in some it may lead to the development of cancer. Even if all known life-style and reproductive factors were to be avoided, it is likely that natural radiation and hereditary factors would still cause some cases of breast cancer.

The ability to recognise specific chromosomal abnormalities in human breast cancer would not only enable us to identify women at high risk but also help to distinguish those breast cancers with a hereditary basis from those occurring randomly. Although specific chromosomal rearrangements have been observed in certain strains of mice which are highly susceptible to breast cancer, no consistent abnormality has so far been observed in women with breast cancer of a familial type. This is in contrast with cancers of the bladder, prostate, lung, bowel, kidney, uterus, ovary and various sarcomas and embryonal tumours, where such biological markers have been shown [9].

Evidence of past virus infection in human breast tissue might also enable us to identify women at high risk to the disease. The role of viruses in the origin of breast cancer is still not clear, although viruses are known to be involved in the initiation of several types of human cancer including those of the liver, uterine cervix, penis and nasopharynx. About 20 years ago, it was suggested that the hereditary basis of human breast cancer might be a virus transmitted from mother to daughter. A recent report [10] has found evidence of retrovirus in the white blood cells of 98% of a group of breast cancer patients. It used to be thought that such a virus might be transmitted in the mother's milk, but against this is the lack of evidence in the human that a maternal family history of breast cancer is any more common that a paternal one. If, how-

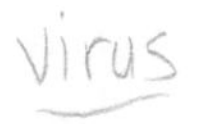

ever, viruses do prove to be an important initiating factor for breast cancer, there is a possibility of immunising women against the infection.

Oncogenes are key growth-control genes which are particularly active in cancer cells. They may become activated either at the point of a chromosomal rearrangement such as described above, as a result of stimulation by chemicals in the environment, or when viruses pass through the cell. While oncogenes are not the cause of cancer, they appear to stimulate the expression of growth factors which play an important role in the malignant behaviour of cells.

A recent finding with considerable promise of application to treatment is that oncogenes have two active portions – one supplies the code for producing particular growth factors and the second is a regulatory section which can turn the mechanism on or off. In the case of breast cancer it has been long been known that natural or synthetic sex hormones can switch the malignant mechanism off, and breast cancer growth can be controlled for 10 or more years in some patients [11]. In the future, cancer cell activity may be inhibited even more effectively, either by using antibodies to block receptors in the cells which take up growth factors, or else by administering specific inhibitory growth factors to counteract the stimulating growth factors [12].

Guidelines for Attempts at Protection

In the future, inhibition of the growth of breast cancer in a women is likely to involve control of oncogene function as outlined above. In the meantime, our first step in protecting a woman against breast cancer is to identify her degree of risk, either from familial susceptibility or other evidence of known risk factors. For the general population, the overall risk of breast cancer might be reduced by avoidance of obesity. For selected women at high risk who are being monitored, one might advise participation in trials of hormonal agents which put the malignant process into a dormant state, or else chemical agents which stop the process advancing from the precancerous state to a fully developed cancer (see Chapter 10).

The rationale of such treatment is based on the knowledge that the origin of any cancer involves two distinct phases. In the first phase or *initiation*, the normal cell is converted into a potentially malignant cell by damage from a virus, chemical or radiation factor, and such damage is irreversible in our present state of knowledge. The second phase of *promotion* is very much longer and involves step-by-step progression of the malignant process until finally cancer manifests clinically. It is these steps which are reversible so that the tumour may be induced to enter a dormant state at any time during its promotion phase. Thus, in our present state of knowledge, an attempt to protect a woman at high risk for breast cancer can mean only an attempt to *delay* the clinical appearance of cancer to the extent that it will permit a normal life expectancy.

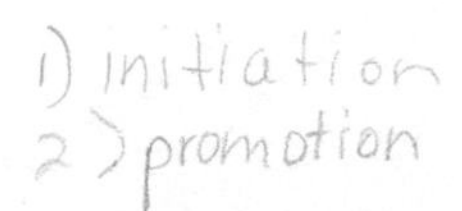

In this context, this means that death from natural causes should occur before the cancer manifests.

In women, hormones from the ovary are almost certainly involved as promoting factors in the progression to invasive cancer (see Chapter 4). Evidence for this is the observation that the risk of a women developing breast cancer is related to the total number of menstrual cycles to which her breasts have been exposed during her life time. (The early onset of menstruation or a late menopause predispose, while pregnancy or an early menopause protect.) Of the ovarian hormones, oestrogen appears to be the major stimulant of cell multiplication and invasion, while there is increasing evidence that progesterone may, under certain circumstances, protect a women against the stimulating effect of oestrogen as a promoter (see Chapter 8).

Other circulating hormones, too, are known to modify the effect of oestrogens on breast tissue, and both androgens and prolactin may affect breast cancer risk in this way. Blood levels of various androgens have been investigated in women with breast cancer but the results are conflicting. However, observations of increased sebaceous gland activity, increased body hair and more masculine build in breast cancer patients suggests that increased male hormone secretion may indeed be a risk factor. It is also well established that Japanese women (who have a very low susceptibility to breast cancer) have relatively low circulating androgen levels.

Recent findings suggest the need for greater investigation of the role of increased androgen levels as a risk factor for breast cancer (see Chapter 4). In a group of women showing increased growth of body hair, 92% were found to have multiple cysts of the ovaries on ultrasound examination although this was not suspected clinically [13]. It is suggested that the elevated levels of androgen found in such women are derived either from the ovaries or adrenal glands, are converted into the oestrogen oestrone and then lead to oversecretion of pituitary hormones such as prolactin and luteinising hormones [14]. It is significant that the cystic changes in the ovaries are similar to those seen in the polycystic ovary syndrome (Stein Leventhal syndrome) which is associated with a *very high risk* of developing breast cancer and shows strong hereditary predisposition. It is interesting, too, that in patients with polycystic ovaries, the increased androgen secretion and excessive body hair can be reduced by the administration of combination type oral contraceptives [14], because of the possibility that the risk of breast cancer may be lessened in the population by these agents (see Chapter 8).

However, it must be recognised that any programme for the protection of the public against breast cancer which is based on long term manipulation of women's hormone balance is likely to be socially unacceptable. Again, attempts at protection based on changing women's life-styles will always be a difficult and incomplete way of coping with the threat of cancer. 'Even if there was a life-style that would reduce cancer rates to 10% of their previous level, it is unlikely that the majority of the public would want to live that way' [15].

The public tends to distinguish sharply between two branches of preventive medicine – what health authorities do to protect them and what they might do themselves to promote their own health. Thus, whereas there is a clamour for health authorities and medical research to intercept all the known causes of cancer (e.g., radiation exposure, industrial carcinogens and food pollutants) the public is less enthusiastic about measures which involve them in avoiding cancer-promoting behaviour. In addition, the advice from health professionals is frequently opposed by commercial interests who may find themselves threatened by campaigns against cancer-promoting habits and life styles.

Because we cannot *promise* the individual women that it will protect her from the danger of breast cancer, it is often difficult to press for a particular life-style such as low fat diet, early pregnancy or prolonged breast feeding. Success would depend not only on how far we can change attitudes in the public but also those among health professionals and governments [16]. Finally, it is often difficult to motivate young women who regard themselves as being healthy and are not particularly concerned about long-term health dangers (a problem typically seen in the case of young smokers).

Education of the public about cancer prevention in general presents specific problems because it is technically complex to explain and arouses deep emotions and fears. People tend to remember information which supports their preconceived notions, and much of the effect of cancer education depends on what the person wishes to know and hear and also on cancer contacts he or she may have had previously. (Several studies confirm that fear of an illness is increased with the individual's personal acquaintance with some suffering from it.) In addition, cancer education may be *counterproductive* if it is confined to giving people knowledge about recognising the disease, without convincing them at the same time that they will benefit if they seek treatment earlier (see Chapter 11).

For example, one early study [17] showed that women who knew that their symptoms indicated breast cancer delayed visiting their doctors more than did those who were genuinely ignorant of the significance of their symptoms. Yet a subsequent study, after a public education campaign in the area, showed that those who reported most promptly were those more likely to know the advantage of early diagnosis and treatment. If women regard themselves as at risk but can see no positive and useful action to take, they take refuge in denial, while relatives of breast cancer patients are more likely to seek early treatment if they have previously received an explanation of the nature of the disease and the purpose of treatment [18].

In spite of this, it is important for women to receive education on breast cancer prevention or screening when they attend their general practitioners for other reasons (such as illness or injury), since they are unlikely to go to their doctors specifically to enquire about changing their life-styles. Unfortunately, the training of physicians in preventive medicine tends to be deficient. Medical education concentrates more on high-tech treatment of acute illness, and lack of time deters most physicians from talking about preventive measures with patients who are not only reluctant to accept them but cannot be *guaranteed* personal benefit from observing them.

Reservations about Screening Programmes

It has recently become clear that breast cancer disseminates to distant sites at a very early stage in the development of the disease. By the time the primary tumour is palpable in the breast, the majority of cases have already spread through the blood stream, although many patients will survive 30 years or longer before these distant metastases become clinically apparent [19]. This finding has led to a search for methods of diagnosing the localised cancer before it is palpable.

Mass screening of the population for early cancer is based on the premise that early detection of an established cancer will lead to a higher survival rate than if the disease were allowed to develop until it became obvious to the patient. Positive evidence of such an ability is available only in the case of two cancers so far – cancer of the breast and cancer of the bowel. While screening leads to a lower mortality rate also in the case of cervical cancer, it is due to the ability to diagnose a *precursor* of the cancer.

In the case of cancer of the breast, the higher survival rate found in screened cases does not necessarily prove that more cancers are being cured. One would expect to find a higher 5 or 10 year survival rate in patients whose cancers were found by screening when compared with similar cancers found by the patient. This is because the former are being diagnosed earlier in the natural history of the disease and the resulting increased duration of survival is referred to as 'lead time' (see Chapter 9).

While trials of population screening for breast cancer claim that survival rates can be increased by up to 30% in the screened group, the guidelines for conducting such screening are still not agreed. An American review has concluded that 'nation-wide screening for breast cancer is desirable although at the present time we have insufficient data to select either entrance ages, periodicity or use of risk factors' [20]. So far, two studies have shown significantly improved survival rates amongst women over the age of 50, taking part in mass screening programmes. Screening series may yield short-term but not long-term increases in survival rates and proof of additional cures may have to wait another 20 or 30 years of follow up. About 20% of cancers discovered at screening already show evidence of spread to the axillary nodes, suggesting that current methods of screening still cannot detect tumours sufficiently early to guarantee cure.

Thus, screening programmes for breast cancer need constant re-evaluation in order to determine their true value. Nevertheless, whether or not more breast cancers are being cured, earlier diagnosis offers an increased possibility of less extensive surgery, because breast conservation and radiation treatment is being increasingly used in the treatment of *small* tumours (see Chapter 9). These arguments about the value of screening have to be considered very carefully by third world nations who have to consider the priority of breast cancer screening as against other health measures which may yield a greater health return for the same expenditure.

Reservations about public cancer screening programmes need to be expressed also because recent publicity in the media may have created public expectations which are too high in relation to the cancerophobia they may cause (see Chapter 11). Even the normal anxiety induced by breast self-examination may not always be justified by its results. It is argued that women who find non-symptomatic benign lumps in the breast by self-examination are exposed to unnecessary anxiety, unnecessary medical investigation (even including surgery), and those not finding such lumps are subject to the risk of false reassurance. Below the age of 30 or 35, false positive findings so greatly outnumber self-detected cancers, that breast self-examination may do more harm than good [21].

Comparing Costs of Screening and Protection

It is important for Western countries to revise the low priority being given to research programmes for protection against cancer. Options must be examined so that the money which is spent will provide the maximum of benefit. Since we have shown that earlier detection may not eradicate breast cancer but merely reduce its short term mortality rate, it suggests that a higher proportion of health resources should be spent on investigating protection of some women at risk by hormonal, dietary or chemical means.

There is growing evidence that low dose oestrogen/progestogen replacement therapy may protect postmenopausal women against breast cancer and that certain formulations of combined type oral contraceptives may at the same time reduce the risk of breast cancer in premenopausal women. Surprisingly, almost no biological research in suitable models is being carried out to establish the optimal formulations (see Chapter 8).

It is important also to keep the costs of cancer screening in proportion, relative to the rest of expenditure on health care. It has been calculated that if all types of current cancer screening available were to be applied annually to all individuals over 40 in the USA, it would consume 10–15% of all money spent on health care. It would cost twice as much as the present cost of treating all cancer patients, and might eliminate between one tenth and one third of cancer mortality, extending the average person's life by about 6 months [5]. As finances are not limitless, we must look for the most effective way to use the money spent on cancer control.

Various obstacles prevent screening programmes making a major impact on cancer control. In the case of lung cancer, screening is relatively expensive and the finding of earlier disease does not necessarily ensure additional cures (as is the case for breast cancer screening). In the case of cervical cancer, the potential for reducing the mortality of the disease is considerable, but the problem is to get those women most at risk to take part in screening programmes. Thus, not only is cancer screening an expensive use of health resources but also it fails to eradicate the disease and needs to be applied repeatedly in order to maintain its effectiveness. Increasing the frequency of screening may increase the return, but a point is reached where considerable increase in costs yields only a minimal increase in earlier diagnosis.

We need to subject breast screening programmes to a cost–benefit analysis if we are to judge whether the benefits outweigh the cost of not conducting such a service. (Every society has to decide health priorities according to its economic ability, and in Western countries such value judgements are made every day in relation to every type of medical expenditure.) In Canada, it has been calculated that for every 50 women who have annual mammograms for 5 years, *one year of life is potentially gained* in a breast cancer patient [22]. (This is based on the assumption that the age of 70 is the mean life expectation in normal women.) In the UK it has been calculated that the cost is greater, and that it requires 100 women to have annual mammograms for 20 years to potentially gain one year of life in a patient [23]. For women aged between 40 and 49, about ten times as many women would need to be screened for similar benefit as that in older women.

It is at present impossible to compare the *cost effectiveness* of screening with that of prevention in the case of breast cancer, because we are at present unable to specify a measure protecting against cancer which could be recommended to *all* women, apart possibly from avoiding obesity. Each woman's choice of a specific measure to protect her against breast cancer will depend on how far she values the possible advantages against the disadvantages, and one woman might make a different choice to another. The state also has a dilemma because of political pressures. A public screening programme for breast cancer is said to potentially gain 3 months' life expectancy for the average women, while it would be many years before a research programme on protection against breast cancer could be proved to show benefit. Protective measures would also require unpopular self-control action by the public, similar to the anti-smoking measures demanded in the case of lung cancer prevention.

Lung cancer provides an example of the cost-effectiveness of prevention versus that of screening. It has been calculated that if lung cancer could be eliminated, it would increase the life expectancy of the average male smoker by about 1.5 years. The results of screening programmes for this disease are not encouraging and it is calculated that intensive screening by X-rays and sputum examination every four months might increase the life expectancy of a smoker by about 40 days [5]. On the other hand, if the cost of such a screening programme were used for an education programme to convince smokers to stop smoking, the cost per year of life saved would be less than 1% of that involved in a screening programme. This calculation considers only the improvement of life expectancy from reducing lung cancer risk, but there would be a further improvement from decreasing the incidence of other tobacco-induced lung and heart conditions.

Conclusion

The selection of a monitoring or protection programme for a women who is at high risk to breast cancer involves personal value judgements both by the women and by the physician who is advising her. There is no one correct decision, because it depends on what value is attached by a women to the outcome in relation to the problems or anxieties involved in the monitoring or protection programme. Which is better, a complicated anxiety-producing programme which has a good chance of reducing a woman's risk, or a less complex programme which has only a fair chance? What is best for one women may not necessarily be best for another, and physicians and counsellors must help each women find a programme which fits in best with her personal needs.

References

1. Bailar, J.C., Smith, E.M. (1986). Progress against cancer. *N. Engl. J. Med.,* **314**, 1226–1232.
2. Silman, A.J. (1987). Recent trends in cancer in England and Wales. *Cancer Care in Medical Education,* 10–14.
3. Mettlin, C. (1987). End results, interhospital differences and trends in patterns of care for gynecologic cancer. *Cancer,* **60**, 1695–1699.
4. Stoll, B.A. (1986). Components of a prognostic index. In Stoll, B.A. (ed.), *Breast Cancer: Treatment and Prognosis*, Blackwell Scientific, Oxford, 115–131.
5. Eddy, D.M. (1984). The economics of cancer prevention and detection. *Cancer,* **47**, 1200–1209.
6. Lynch, H.T., Albano, W.A., Danes, B.S. *et al.* (1984). Genetic predisposition to breast cancer. *Cancer,* **53**, 612–622.
7. Mulvihill, J.J. (1977). Genetic repertory of human neoplasia. In Mulvihill, J.J., Miller, B.W., Fraumeni, J.F., (eds), *Genetics of Human Cancer*, Raven Press, New York, 137–143.
8. Kozak, F.K., Hall, J.G., Baird, P.A. (1986). Familial breast cancer in males. *Cancer,* **58**, 2736–2739.
9. Sandberg, A.A., Turc-Carel, C. (1987). The cytogenetics of solid tumours. *Cancer,* **59**, 387–395.
10. Al Sumidae, A.M., Leinster, S.J., Hart, C.A., *et al.* (1988). Particles with properties of retrovirus in monocytes from patients with breast cancer. *Lancet,* **i**, 5–9.
11. Stoll, B.A. (1988). Combination endocrine therapy. In Stoll, B.A., (ed.) *Endocrine Management of Breast Cancer: Contemporary Therapy*, S. Karger, Basel, 80–101.
12. Sainsbury, J.R.C. (1988). Growth factors and their receptors as mediators of response. In Stoll, B.A. (ed.) *Endocrine Management of Cancer: Biological Bases*, S. Karger, Basel, 35–44.

13. Polson, D.W., Adams, J., Wadsworth, J., Franks, S. (1988). Polycystic ovaries – a common finding in normal women. *Lancet*, **i**, 870–872.
14. McKenna, T.J. (1988). Pathogenesis and treatment of polycystic ovary syndrome. *N. Engl. J. Med.*, **318**, 558–562.
15. Baltimore, D. (1987). The impact of the discovery of oncogenes on cancer mortality rates will come slowly. *Cancer*, **59**, 1985–1986.
16. Mettlin, C., Cummings, K.M. (1982). Communication and behavior change for cancer control. In Mettlin, C. and Murphy, G.P., (eds), *Issues in Cancer Screening and Communications*, Alan R. Liss, New York, 135–150.
17. Aitken-Swan, J., Paterson, R. (1955). The cancer patient; delay in seeking advice. *Brit. Med. J.*, **1**, 623–636.
18. Cobb, B., Clark, R., McGuire, C., Howe, C.D. (1954). Patient-responsible delay of treatment in breast cancer. *Cancer*, **7**, 920–925.
19. Hibberd, A.D. (1986). Surgery: prolonged survival or cure. In Stoll, B.A. (ed.), *Breast Cancer – Treatment and Prognosis*, Blackwell Scientific, Oxford, 3–12.
20. Carlile, T., Hadaway, E. (1985). Screening for breast cancer. In Stoll, B.A. (ed.), *Screening and Monitoring of Cancer*, John Wiley, Chichester, 135–152.
21. Frank, J.W., Mai, V. (1985). Breast self-examination in young women. *Lancet*, **ii**, 654–657.
22. Miller, A.B. (1982). Screening for cancer of the cervix and breast. In Mettlin, C. and Murphy, G.P. (eds), *Issues in Cancer Screening and Communications*, Alan R. Liss, New York, 41–54.
23. Moss, S., Chamberlain, J., Ellman, R. (1987). Breast cancer screening. *Lancet*, **i**, 1153–1154.

Chapter 2

Effect of Race, Geography and Social Class

CURTIS METTLIN and ELINOR R. SCHOENFELD

Race, geography and social class may interact in a complex way in influencing the risk of developing breast cancer. Different regions of the world are populated by different racial groups and may also vary in their levels of economic development. Within a specific region, different racial groups may have different social class distributions. The reasons for examining these distributions are first, that higher prevalence of cancer in one region may indicate the need for suitable preventive programs. Secondly, variations within a region according to race or social class may suggest the need to target a specific group with a cancer control program tailored to its degree of risk. Finally, variations in risk between persons and places can reflect factors which are important in breast cancer development, and this knowledge can help us to control the disease.

Patterns of Distribution

International comparisons of incidence rates are difficult to evaluate because they involve many registries reporting data with different degrees of completeness for different years of study. Mortality data, in contrast, tend to be more uniformly collected and are available for several continuous years.

Figure 1 shows selected age-adjusted mortality rates for cancer of the breast [1]. That Asian women have the lowest rates of breast cancer mortality in the world is reflected in the low rate reported for Japan. Although not shown, the Chinese in Hong Kong and Singapore similarly have deaths rates which are one third (or less) those of comparably aged women in the United Kingdom or the United States. Other sources suggest that low incidence rates are observed for Indian women in Bombay [2].

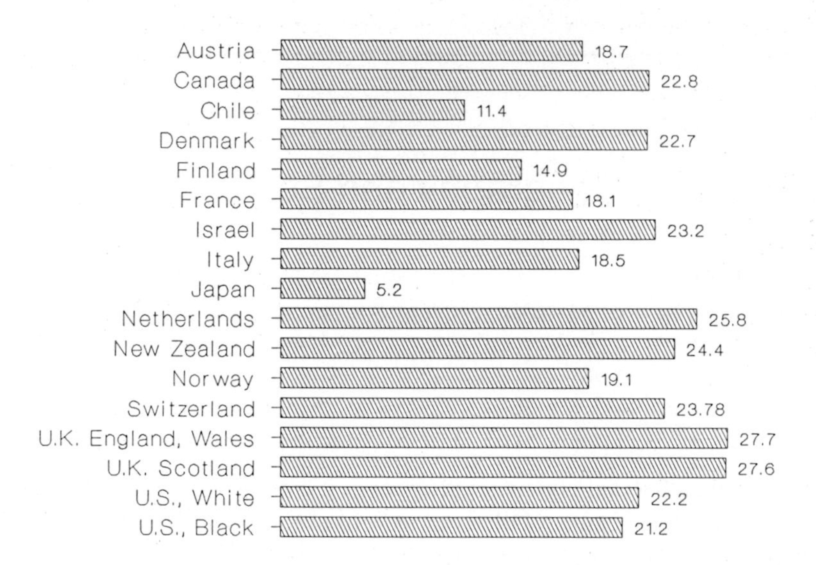

Figure 1 Age-adjusted mortality from breast cancer in selected nations, 1978–9, rate per 100 000. Source: ref [1].

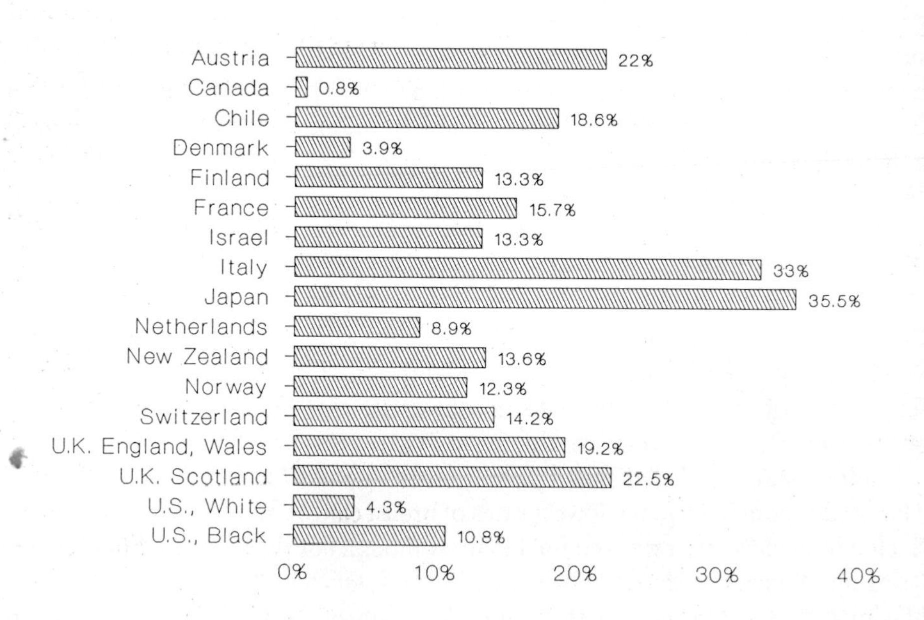

Figure 2 Percent change in age-adjusted mortality from breast cancer 1958–9 to 1978–9. Source: ref [1].

In Israel, the non-Jewish population exhibits low incidence whereas the population of Jewish women has a rate comparable to those of European populations.

Figure 2 shows the percent change in age-adjusted breast cancer mortality rates between 1958–9 and 1978–9 for the same selected nations, and it appears that some of the areas which have had the lowest rates are experiencing the greatest change. Although remaining low compared to Western regions, a clearly rising trend is evident in Japan where there are also parallel increases in the mortality rates for ovary and prostate cancers [3]. In countries where mortality has been high, only marginal levels of increase are observed. For example, among whites in the United States, the mortality data suggest little change in incidence although this inference may be misleading. Recent data [4] do suggest that breast cancer incidence in the United States is rising but may not be reflected in the mortality data because of improved results from breast cancer treatment.

Figure 1 shows that black women in the United States have a slightly lower overall breast cancer mortality rate compared to white women but comparison of the overall figures masks some important differences. The advantage of black women with respect to breast cancer risk is true only for the population over forty, while under age forty the incidence of breast cancer is similar to that of white women and the mortality rate is actually higher. Overall, the difference in mortality rates between US blacks and whites appears to have narrowed recently, and it has been suggested that women born after 1925 tend to bear the same risk regardless of race [5].

Large portions of the racially diverse United States population are monitored by the Surveillance, Epidemiology, and End Results (SEER) program of the US National Cancer Institute. Figure 3 shows the breast cancer incidence rates for different racial and ethnic groups residing in the United States [6]. Whites and Hawaiians have the highest rates, with persons of Asian, Hispanic, and American Indian descent having the lowest incidence rates.

The lower risk for persons of Asian descent in the United States has been further confirmed by a study of cancer patterns in four ethnic groups in Hawaii relative to the rates of mainland whites. It found the highest breast cancer incidence ratios among Hawaiians followed in order by Chinese, Japanese and Filipino women [7]. Again, while some cancers, such as those of lung and colon, have tended to rise among the Chinese in the United States above the levels observed in Taiwan, the United States Chinese women continue to have breast cancer rates which are as low as the Taiwanese [8].Other studies of populations migrating east across the Pacific have shown the relative importance of regional as opposed to racial origin as a risk factor for breast carcinoma. Three decades ago, breast cancer death rates among Japanese-American women were nearer the rates in Japan than those of white women in the United States. By 1970, however, the rates among Japanese-American women in San Francisco has risen substantially, so that they more closely approximated those of whites [9]. This was particularly true for persons of Japanese ancestry born in the

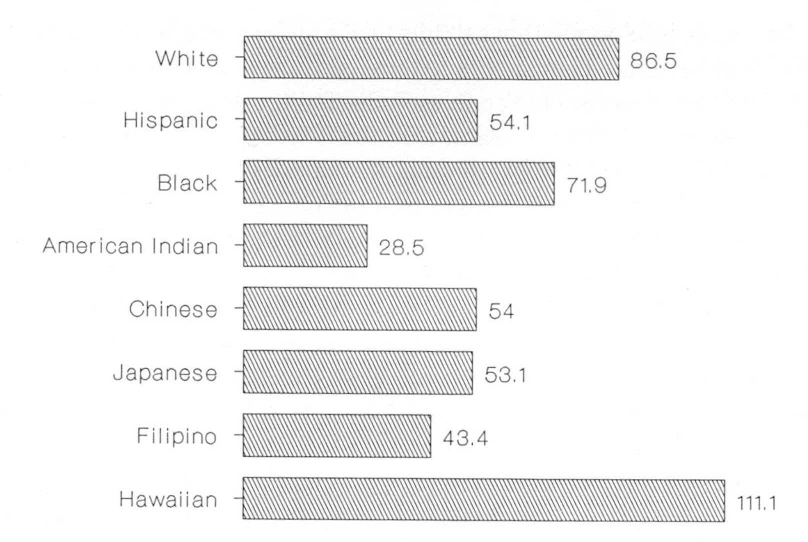

Figure 3. Age-adjusted incidence of breast cancer in different population groups in the United States, 1978–81, rate per 100 000. Source: ref [6].

United States, but increases in rates were also evident among Americans who were born in Japan. The tendency for breast cancer rates in migrating populations to accommodate to the prevailing levels in the host population had been observed previously in the case of Polish migrants to the United States [10].

The observation noted above that the rates of breast cancer among Chinese-American women have not increased over the homeland levels [8] may not be in conflict with the general pattern of increasing breast cancer risk among Asian migrant populations to the United States. MacMahon and colleagues [11] have observed that the change in breast cancer risk among Japanese-Americans trailed behind changes in risk for other tumor types such as cancers of the colon and lung. Colon and lung cancer risk has already increased among Chinese-Americans and this suggests that the acculturation process will eventually lead to a higher breast cancer mortality.

Effect of Race and Geography

The fact that breast cancer risk changes as populations migrate is evidence that a substantial part of that risk is not determined by genetic predisposition. The wide distribution of breast cancer as a major problem suggests also that it is not the result of localized environmental carcinogens. With the exception of the known risk of radiation-induced cancer, the overall epidemiological picture suggests that much of the risk of breast cancer is culturally mediated and that groups and populations modify their risk as they acquire or abandon the practices and habits which constitute the risk factors for the disease.

The most commonly noted cultural practice which correlates to some extent with both race and place of residence is diet (see Chapter 6). While not all the data agree that dietary fat enhances breast cancer risk, the international differences in rates do support such a hypothesis. Rose and colleagues [3] have related the 1978–9 mortality rates for cancers of the breast, prostate, ovary and colon in different nations to 1979–81 food availability data. They observed strong correlations between animal fat consumption and breast cancer mortality, particularly for postmenopausal breast cancer. They observed also that increasing rates of dietary fat availability corresponded to increasing breast cancer rates in several countries. That the type of fat used may be important was suggested by data showing that regions which had high vegetable fat consumption (such as olive oil) did not have correspondingly high breast cancer rates.

Japan also shows a correlation between the recently increased consumption of Western-style fat-rich foods (such as butter and margarine, cheese, ham and sausage) and increased age-adjusted death rates for breast and ovarian cancer, and a lag-time of ten years is suggested between the change in dietary habits and the change in disease risk [12]. Another study in Japan examined diets of the husbands of Japanese women who had breast cancer compared to men whose wives did not have the disease (on the assumption that the men's diets reflected the spouses' exposures) and observed a higher consumption of high-fat foods such as beef, butter and sausage among the husbands of breast cancer patients [13].

However, one cannot necessarily conclude that dietary fat is of singular importance in breast cancer etiology [14] nor that it explains the regional and racial differences. For example, age at menarche, age at first full-term pregnancy, and age at menopause are all established risk factors for breast cancer among Caucasian women and case-control studies in Hawaii have shown that these risk factors apply also to breast cancer among Japanese women [15]. Women with breast cancer in Japan and the United States have been compared with respect to all of these factors, and although the parous Japanese women do exhibit a later age at first birth, higher rates of nulliparity and later age at menarche were found [16]. The investigators estimated that even the later age at menarche alone could result in as much as 50% lower breast cancer rate in Japan compared to the United States.

Recently, the age at menarche in Japan has been decreasing, a trend that may be associated with the increasing breast cancer risk. The increased risk among Japanese migrants to the United States may also be associated with factors other than Western dietary habits. The female offspring of migrant Japanese women have been shown to be less likely to be nulliparous and more likely to bear children before age 20 compared to the first generation of migrants [9]. Both these trends would be expected to increase the risk to Japanese-American women and this has apparently occurred.

Differences in exposure to ovarian and reproductive risk factors may also explain the differences in risk between black and white women in the United States. One study examined the effects of educational attainment, age at menarche, age at first childbirth and age at menopause in both black and white breast cancer patients compared to race-matched controls [5]. Similar effects for these risk factors were observed among both race groups. A similar but substantially larger study of risk factors among black breast cancer patients and controls found late age at first birth, early age of menarche and nulliparity all to be associated with increased risk of breast cancer [17]. It also observed that a history of benign breast disease and family history of breast cancer led to a higher risk of breast cancer.

While similar risk factors may operate in both black and white women, the latter may have greater exposure to these factors. It is reported that white women in the United States tend to have a later age at first live birth compared to blacks and an earlier age of menopause [18]. Both these factors may explain the lower risk among postmenopausal black women. US blacks also have a slightly earlier average age of menarche and this may account for the greater risk among younger black women.

In summary, the data on risk factors among US whites, US blacks, Japanese-American women and Japanese women suggest that breast cancers in these different populations do not have substantially different etiologies. The reproductive and other predisposing factors associated with the disease tend to be similar for all groups but what does appear to differ is the degree to which the populations are exposed to the risk factors. The study of migrating groups suggests that as they adopt similar reproductive patterns and other culturally-determined patterns of living such as diet, differences in risk tend to diminish.

Effect of Socio-Economic Factors

Several types of cancer are related to the socio-economic characteristics of populations and usually it is low social class attainment (as measured by educational level or by income) which is linked to higher cancer risk. Greater exposure to environmental carcinogens, less access to health care and less knowledge about preventive measures, may all play a role in this general tendency. Breast cancer, however, tends not follow the general pattern. A review of twelve studies from the early 1940s to the later 1970s, involving data from Denmark, the United States, Scotland, Norway, Hong Kong, Australia and Finland, showed higher breast cancer rates linked to *higher* social class attainment in all studies [19]. This was true whether incidence or mortality was examined, and whether social class was measured by income, education, occupation or husband's occupation.

In the United States, race and social class are related factors. Devesa and Diamond [20] have attempted to determine the extent that the differences in breast cancer risk between black and white women in the United States are the products of race as opposed to socio-economic differences. They observed that the tendency toward higher risk associated with higher income and higher levels of educational attainment occurred independently of race. Their data suggested that both black and white women with the same socio-economic status were at similar levels of risk, and that much of the difference in disease risk between blacks and whites in the United States could be explained by the effects of educational level and income.

How higher socio-economic attainment translates into higher breast cancer risk is not certain. As with the international variations, the dietary habits associated with socio-economic attainment may affect risk. Animal fat consumption is positively linked to income but there are other class-related differences in exposure to risk. Age at childbearing and rates of nulliparity similarly are linked to social class in a manner that may contribute to the risk differential.

Effect on Prognosis

The SEER data in the United States show some variability in the survival rate for breast cancers occurring among different racial and ethnic groups [21]. Figure 4 shows that some of the groups with a low incidence tend also to have a more favourable long-term prognosis. Asian women have the best survival rates while American Indians and blacks have the poorest. Other data which support the notion that survi-

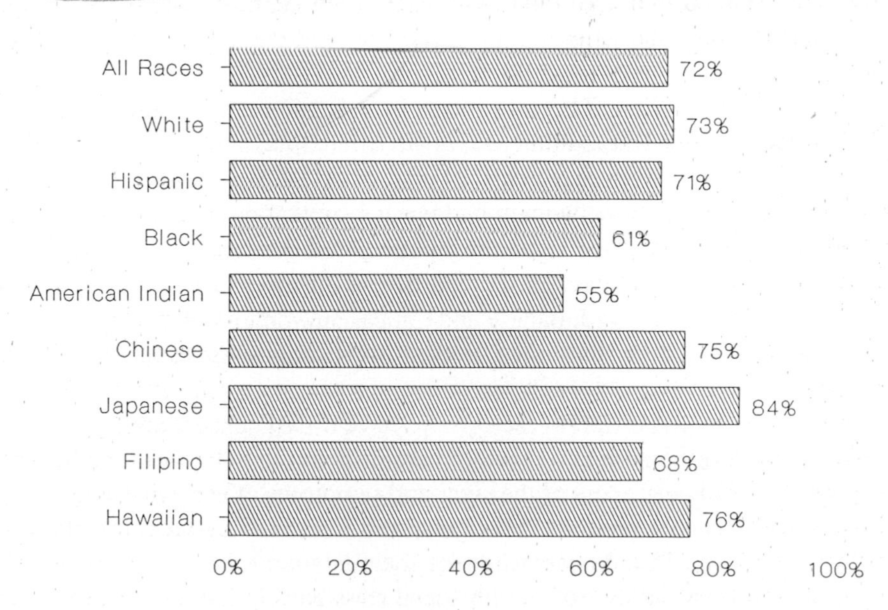

Figure 4 Five-year relative survival in percent for breast cancer in different population groups in the United States, patients diagnosed 1973–81. Source: ref [21].

val rates vary by race are observations of a poorer prognosis among South African blacks compared to whites [22] and a better prognosis for Japanese women in Japan compared to that for whites in the United States [23].

International comparisons of prognosis are difficult to interpret because of variability in criteria for staging, facilities for diagnosis, treatment and follow-up but a large survey of the American College of Surgeons has confirmed that the overall 5-year survival of black patients was explained by the tendency for cancers in black women to be diagnosed at a more advanced stage with greater nodal involvement, and to show evidence of greater biological aggressiveness.

Thus, Leffall [25] has observed that the tumors diagnosed in black women tended to be larger whether the cancer was invasive or non-invasive. (White women with non-invasive carcinoma presented with tumors less than one centimeter diameter in 21.3% of cases compared to only 8.3% of cases among black women.) However, Asian women in the studies proved less likely to die from breast cancer compared to white breast cancer patients, even after adjusting for stage of disease, age at diagnosis and histology. This persistent effect for ethnicity has also been observed among patients in Hawaii [26].

It is uncertain how much the survival differential in black women is the result of differences in medical care and diagnosis as opposed to greater tumor aggressiveness. In the American College of Surgeons studies, some survival differences were present even after stage, histology, patient age and other prognostic factors were considered and this would suggest a biological difference in the tumors. Supporting such a conclusion is the observation that breast cancers among black women show a different histologic spectrum from that in whites [27] and the finding of less well-differentiated tumors among blacks [28].

Microscopic examination of breast cancers from Japanese and Caucasian women treated in Hawaii showed more numerous *in situ* carcinomas and more extensive lymphocytic infiltrates in Japanese women [29]. As would be expected from their more favorable prognosis, Japanese women had fewer lymph node metastases and it was suggested that they might have a genetically-mediated hormonal or immunological susceptibility to disease progression. Comparison of the age and stage-specific breast cancer incidence rates among Japanese and Caucasian women in Japan suggests that post-menopausal cancers may have slower average growth rates in Japanese women [30].

There is no doubt that different race groups have breast cancers diagnosed at different stages of development as a result of inequities in the delivery of medical care or different levels of awareness of the signs and symptoms of early disease. Thus, in a series of breast cancer patients in Virginia, differences in survival for black and white patients became insignificant when the socio-economic level of the patient was considered [31] while patients of similar social class had similar survival regardless of race. Again, in New York State black–white differences by region in the stage of breast cancer at diagnosis were correlated with regional variation in the income differential between blacks and whites [32]. Where the differences between black and white incomes were greatest, so too were the differences in the stage of disease at diagnosis. In contrast, however, a report from Texas showed that race and ethnicity effects on survival persisted even after the effects of socio-economic status, stage of disease and delay in seeking care were taken into account [33].

Conclusion

Studies of breast cancer risk among different social classes and among persons of different racial or national origin have identified ovarian and reproductive risk factors which may explain different patterns of breast cancer incidence and mortality. In addition, international comparisons have helped to identify other possible sources of risk such as diet.The data suggest that the risk of breast cancer is not inherited in a race-linked manner but that persons of different race, national origin or social class exposed to the same risk factors will manifest the disease at similar rates. However, even many years after persons have left their native lands, there is still a variability in incidence. We need to establish the extent to which such differences are the result of differential access to medical care, differences in exposure to risk or biological differences in susceptibility to breast cancer.

References

1. Kurihara, M., Aoki, K., Tominaga, S. (1984). *Cancer Mortality Statistics in the World*, University of Nagoya, Nagoya, Japan.
2. Waterhouse, J., Muir, C., Shanmugaratnam, K., Powell, J. (1982). *Cancer Incidence on Five Continents*, Vol. 4, IARC, Lyon, France.
3. Rose, D.P., Boyar, A.P., Wynder, E.L. (1986). International comparisons of mortality rates for cancer of the breast, ovary, prostate, and colon and per capita food consumption. *Cancer*, **58**, 2263–2371.
4. Devesa, S.S., Silverman, D.T., Young, J.L. Jr, Pollack, E.S., Brown, C.C., Horm, J.W., Percy, C.L., Myers, M.H., McKay, F.W., Fraumeni, J.R. Jr, (1987). Cancer incidence and mortality trends among whites in the United States, 1947–1984. *J. Nat. Cancer Inst.*, **79**, 701–770.
5. Austin, H., Cole, P., Wynder, E.L. (1979). Breast cancer in black American women. *Int. J. Cancer*, **24**, 541–544.
6. Baquet, C.R., Ringen, K., Pollack, E.S., Young, J.L., Horm, J.W., Ries, L.A.G. (1986). *Cancer Among Blacks and Other Minorities: Statistical Profiles*, National Institutes of Health Pub. **86**, 2785.
7. Kolonel, L.N. (1980). Cancer patterns of four ethnic groups in Hawaii. *J. Nat. Cancer Inst.*, **65**, 1127–1139.
8. King, H., Locke, F.B. (1980). Cancer mortality among Chinese in the United States. *J. Nat. Cancer Inst.*, **65**, 1141–1148.

9. Buell, P. (1973) Changing incidence of breast cancer in Japanese-American women. *J. Nat. Cancer Inst.*, **51**, 1479–1483.
10. Staszewski, J., Haenszel, W.M. (1965). Cancer mortality among the Polish-born in the United States. *J. Nat. Cancer Inst.*, **35**, 291–297.
11. MacMahon, B., Cole, P., Brown, J. (1973). Etiology of human breast cancer: a review. *J. Nat. Cancer Inst.*, **50**, 21–42.
12. Kato, I., Tominaga, S., Kuroishi, T. (1987). Relationship between westernization of dietary habits and mortality from breast and ovarian cancers in Japan. *Jpn. J. Cancer Res. (G)*, **78**, 349–357.
13. Nomura, A., Henderson, B.E., Lee, J. (1978). Breast cancer and diet among the Japanese in Hawaii. *Amer. L. Clin. Nutr.*, **31**, 2020–2025.
14. Mettlin, C. (1984). Diet and the epidemiology of human breast cancer. *Cancer*, **53**, 2201–2205.
15. Nomura, A.M., Lee, J., Kolonel, L.N., Hirohata, T. (1984). Breast cancer in two populations with different levels of risk for disease. *Amer. J. Epidem.*, **119**, 496–502.
16. Hoel, D.G., Wakabayashi, T., Pike, M.C. (1983). Secular trends in the distributions of the breast cancer risk factors – menarche, first birth, menopause, and weight-in Hiroshima and Nagasaki, Japan. *Amer. J. Epidem.*, **118**, 78–89.
17. Schatzkin, A., Palmer, J.R., Rosenberg, L., Helmrich, S.P., Miller, D.R., Kaufman, D.W., Lesko, S.M., Shapiro, S. (1987). Risk factors for breast cancer in black women. *J. Nat. Cancer Inst.,* **78**, 213–217.
18. Gray, G.E., Henderson, B.E., Pike, M.C. (1980). Changing ratio of breast cancer incidence rates with age of black females compared with white females in the United States. *J. Nat. Cancer Inst.*, **64**, 461–463
19. Logan, W.P.D. (1982). *Cancer Mortality by Occupation and Social Class, 1851–1971.* IARC Sci. Publ. No. 36.
20. Devesa, S., Diamond, E.L. (1980). Association of breast cancer and cervical cancer incidences with income and education among whites and blacks. *J. Nat. Cancer Inst.*, **65**, 515–528.
21. Young, J.L. Jr, Ries, L.G., Pollack, E.S. (1984). Cancer patient survival among ethnic groups in the United States. *J. Nat. Cancer Inst.*, **73**, 341–352.
22. Walker, A.R.P., Walker, B.F., Tshabalala, E.N., Isaacson, C., Segal, I. (1984). Low survival of South African urban black women with breast cancer. *Brit. J. Cancer*, **49**, 241–244.
23. Wynder, E.L., Kajitani, T., Kuno, J., Lucas, J.C. Jr, DePalo, A., Farrow, J. (1963). A comparison of survival rates between American and Japanese patients with breast cancer. *Surg. Gynec. Obstet.*, **117**, 196–200.
24. Natarajan, N., Nemoto, T., Mettlin, C., Murphy, G.P. (1985). Race-related differences in breast cancer patients: results of the 1982 national survey of breast cancer by the American College of Surgeons. *Cancer*,**56**, 1704–1709.
25. Leffall, L.D. (1981). Breast cancer in black women. *Ca.-A. Cancer J. for Physicians*, **31**, 209–211.
26. LeMarchard, L., Kolonel, L.N., Nomnura, A.M.Y. (1984). Relationship of ethnicity and other prognostic factors to breast cancer survival patterns in Hawaii. *J. Nat. Cancer Inst.*, **73**, 1259–1265.
27. Mohla, S., Sampson, C.D., Khan, T., Enterline, J.P., Leffall, L. Jr, White, J.E., Gabriel, B.W., Hunter, J.B. (1982). Estrogen and progesterone receptors in breast cancer in black Americans: correlation of receptor data with tumor differentiation. *Cancer*, **50**, 552–559.
28. Ownby, H.E., Fredrick, J., Russo, J., Brooks, S.C., Swanson, G.M., Heppner, G.H., Brennan, M.J. (1985). Racial differences in breast cancer patients. *J. Nat. Cancer Inst.*, **75**, 55–60.
29. Stemmermann, G.N., Catts, A., Fukunaga, F.H., Horie, A., Nomura, A.M.Y. (1985). Breast cancer in women of Japanese and Caucasian ancestry in Hawaii. *Cancer*, **56**, 206–209.

30. Ward-Hinds, M., Kolonel, L.N., Nomura, A.M.Y., Lee, J. (1982). Stage-specific breast cancer incidence rates by age among Japanese and Caucasian women in Hawaii, 1960–1979. *Brit. J. Cancer*, **45**, 118–123.
31. Dayal, H.H., Power, R.N., Chiu, C. (1982). Race and socio-economic status in survival from breast cancer. *J. Chron. Dis.*, **35**, 675–683.
32. Polednak, A.P. (1986). Breast cancer in black and white women in New York State: case distribution and incidence rates by clinical stage at diagnosis. *Cancer*, **58**, 807–815.
33. Vernon, S.W., Tilley, B.C., Neale, A.V., Steinfeldt, L. (1985). Ethnicity, survival, and delay in seeking treatment for symptoms of breast cancer. *Cancer*, **55**, 1563–1571.

Chapter 3

Familial and Genetic Factors – New Evidence

HENRY T. LYNCH, JOSEPH N. MARCUS, PATRICE WATSON and
JANE F. LYNCH

Breast cancer is a major health problem and cause of anxiety in the United States [1] and in discussing familial breast cancer (FBC) and hereditary breast cancer (HBC), it is important that these terms be clearly defined. FBC and HBC are commonly used interchangeably by authors to describe clustering of breast cancer among the relatives of a breast cancer patient. However, it is essential to distinguish between the terms 'familial' and 'hereditary' when describing families where two or more relatives manifest breast cancer.

Familial or Hereditary?

In the case of familial breast cancer (FBC) we are inferring that the clustering in the particular family could be due to common environmental factors possibly interacting with genetic factors. Since breast cancer is a common disease, chance undoubtedly accounts for many of these familial clusterings which are defined as a patient with two or more primary or secondary relatives with breast cancer. Investigators from all parts of the world have examined the significance of familial aggregations of breast cancer [2, 3] and most agree that the presence of breast cancer in a first degree relative increases a woman's risk of developing breast cancer by 2–3 fold [4].

Sattin *et al.* [5] found that the relative risk (RR) to a woman with an affected first degree relative was 2.3; to women with an affected second degree relative, it was 1.5; and to women with both an affected mother and sister, the RR was 14. Ottman *et al.* [6] studied breast cancer risk to sisters of breast cancer patients in a population-based series of patients diagnosed in Los Angeles county between 1971 and 1975 and observed that sisters of patients with bilateral breast cancer diagnosed at 50 years or younger had an RR = 5 and the risk was even greater for sisters of bilateral cases diagnosed at age 40 years or younger (RR = 10.5). Sisters of unilateral breast cancer patients diagnosed at 50 years or younger did not show a significantly increased breast cancer risk. However, sisters of unilateral cases diagnosed at age 40 years or younger had an RR = 2.4. These studies clearly indicate the existence of families in the general population which show a predisposition to breast cancer.

These epidemiological studies of risk associated with a positive family history have not assumed any specific type of genetic mechanism to account for these results. However, one approach has assumed that some of the familial aggregation was caused by segregation of major breast cancer susceptibility genes [7].

Hereditary breast cancer (HBC) is not a single disease, but a heterogeneous group of breast cancer-prone disorders. It may form part of multiple tumor associations or rarely be associated with cutaneous signs, as in the cancer-associated genodermatosis known as Cowden's disease [2]. Its heterogeneity is of particular importance with respect to tumor variation [2, 8–10], age at onset [11, 12], and risk to the contralateral breast [13]. HBC also may *not* be influenced by commonly accepted risk factors such as age at first pregnancy [14].

Hereditary breast cancer shows certain characteristics in the natural history of the disease [2, 8–11]. These include the following: (a) patients with HBC show a significantly earlier age of onset when compared to the sporadic form [2, 15]; (b) tumor variation and excess of multiple primary cancer, including bilateral breast cancer excess, occurs in specific breast cancer-prone families. The association of multiple tumors may involve cancers of breast and ovary [9] or Sarcoma, Breast cancer, brain tumors, Lung and laryngeal cancer, leukemia, lymphoma, and Adrenal cortical carcinoma (SBLA syndrome) [16, 17]; (c) autosomal dominant mode of genetic transmission [8, 18]; (d) improved survival in HBC patients when compared, stage for stage, with the American College of Surgeons' Audit Series [19].

New knowledge has emerged recently showing in the case of HBC: (a) an extremely early age of onset type; (b) an apparent excess of medullary carcinoma of the breast and a high mitotic index in HBC as compared to sporadic cases; (c) evidence that it accounts for about 9% of the total breast cancer burden and thus requires education of at-risk patients and their physicians.

These aspects are discussed in the rest of this chapter.

Frequency of Familial and Hereditary Breast Cancer

In a consecutive series of patients with histologically verified breast cancer in our Oncology Clinic, we assessed the frequency of sporadic, familial and hereditary types [20]. Figure 1 depicts the change in relative frequency of the respective categories following an intensive follow up of the original cohort of 225 consecutive breast cancer patients. This updated cohort plus 103 new patients revealed that 68% of 328 cases studied were sporadic, 23% were familial, and 9% were hereditary [21].

In most circumstances, the modified nuclear pedigree (Figure 2) will provide suf-

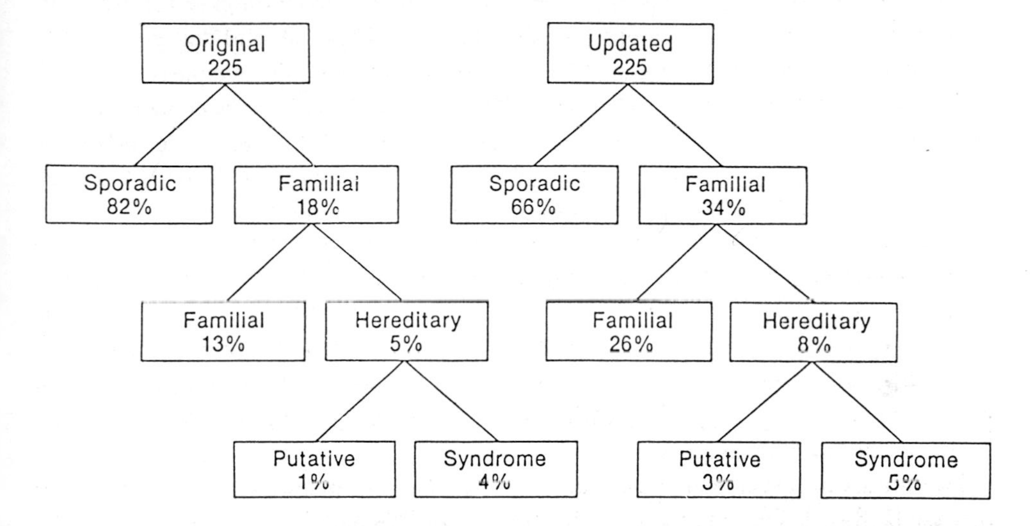

Figure 1 Schematic depicting frequency of sporadic, familial, and hereditary breast cancer as originally documented in a consecutively ascertained series of patients and with findings (updated) after intensive follow up of these same patients. (Reproduced with permission from H.T. Lynch and J.F. Lynch, (1986). *Ca. Genet. Cytogenet.*, **22**,369–71.

Figure 2 Diagram portraying a modified nuclear pedigree, the minimum information needed to evaluate cancer family history. (Reproduced with permission from H.T. Lynch *et al.* (1984). *Surv. Dig. Dis.*, **2**, 244–260.

In most circumstances, the modified nuclear pedigree (Figure 2) will provide sufficient information to enable assessment of the significance of familial or hereditary factors. Note that attention is given to all first degree relatives comprising the patient's siblings, progeny, and parents. Included also are second degree relatives, including both sets of grandparents, aunts, and uncles. These second degree relatives are highly informative in that, being older, they will more likely have passed through the cancer risk age and thus will have shown the pertinent hereditary cancers, should they exist. Both sets of grandparents are important also, because *paternal* transmission (due to the autosomal pattern of inheritance of breast cancer) will be missed if one fails to probe in depth the *paternal* as well as the *maternal* lineage.

Age at Onset in HBC

One of the characteristic features of HBC is a tendency for diagnoses to occur earlier in life. While the mean age at diagnosis in large, unselected series of breast cancer cases is nearly 60, cases from HBC families have a mean age of onset in their mid-40s. As a result, it has been recommended that women from HBC families initiate surveillance earlier in life than is generally recommended, with full surveillance including baseline mammography starting by age 25. Nevertheless, there is great variability in the age at first diagnosis in HBC cases and they may be diagnosed in women in their early 20s (exceedingly rare), more commonly in the premenopausal age group and to a more limited extent, postmenopausally.

Surveillance would be easier if we could predict the age at which the patient is likely to develop breast cancer. For example, if we could identify a subgroup of HBC cases where breast cancer risk is high in *young* adulthood, we could advise these women to begin surveillance even before age 25. By doing so, we could detect the developing cancers in an *early* and more treatable state. On the other hand, if we could identify a subgroup of HBC cases where breast cancer risk is low in young adulthood but high in the perimenopasual or postmenopausal years, we could postpone the initiation of full surveillance until age 35 or 40. By doing so, we could reduce the cost of surveillance and avoid the compliance problems that attend very long surveillance programs.

Clinical observations suggested to us that there may be heterogeneity in the age of onset of cancer among HBC families. While certain families showed a consistent tendency for very early onset breast cancer, other families showed consistently late ages of onset. There were also many examples of families with a wide range of ages at time of diagnosis. In a consecutive series of 328 breast cancer cases studied at the Creighton Oncology Clinic, we found [15] that 112 had a family history of breast cancer in sisters, mothers, aunts, or grandmothers. Thirty of these had been classified as HBC, and the remainder as 'familial' breast cancer [21]. We found that the

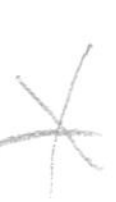

HBC group was heterogeneous with respect to age at diagnosis of breast cancer: young patients (diagnosed before age 40) were more likely to have relatives with early breast cancer diagnoses (age < 40) than were older patients ($p < .001$).

Biological Markers in HBC

Biological markers would be useful if they identified HBC family members at risk or distinguished the hereditary tumor type from its sporadic counterpart. Unfortunately, no sensitive or specific biomarker answering either of these needs currently exists. Ultimately, linkage analysis with specific DNA markers on chromosomes will predict which HBC family members will develop breast cancer.

Histopathology

Certain features in benign breast lesions increase the risk for subsequent development of breast cancer. Proliferative disease with *atypical hyperplasia* constitutes 3–4% of benign breast biopsies [22–24] and is associated with a 4.4–fold increased risk of developing breast cancer. However, when a family history is present (defined as mother, sisters, or daughters with breast cancer), the risk increases to roughly 9–fold. *Juvenile papillomatosis*, characterized by florid intraductal papillomatosis in young women, is a special type of hyperplasia recently described by Rosen *et al.* [25]. There is some suggestion that the small percentage of juvenile papillomatosis patients who concurrently or subsequently develop *in situ* or invasive carcinoma have a more significant family history of breast carcinoma.

Although tumor pathology is not a diagnostic marker in FBC, or HBC, Lagios *et al.* [26] found that 6/15 of patients with tubular carcinoma had a positive family history of breast cancer compared to 31/186 of those with carcinomas lacking tubular history ($p < 0.05$). Other studies have indicated an excess of *medullary carcinoma* in FBC or HBC. Anderson [27] found an increase in this histology in patients with sisters, but not mothers, with breast cancer. Rosen *et al.* [28] observed that women with medullary carcinoma are more likely to have mothers with breast cancer. All these studies concerned FBC.

Studying HBC, Mulcahy and Platt [29] observed excess medullary carcinoma, with or without lymphoid stroma, as compared to sporadic breast cancer (SBC) controls (12/75 *vs* 2/52; $p < 0.05$). We have performed a double-blinded case/control study of breast cancer histopathology from HBC cases, using age-matched and race-matched SBC controls [30]. (Age matching is important since both medullary carcinoma and HBC are known to occur with higher frequencies at younger ages.) While we confirmed an excess of either 'typical' or 'atypical' medullary carcinoma as defined by Ridolfi *et al.* [31] without age matching criteria in force, we did not observe a clear

Proliferative characteristics

Marcus *et al.* [30] noted an increased mitotic grade i.e., higher malignancy) in HBC as compared to SBC (22/35 mitotic grades II and III in HBC *vs* 11/33 in SBC, not age-matched, $p < 0.02$). Since only infiltrating ductal type carcinomas were scored, the result is independent of the effect of the presence of any excess medullary carcinoma, which has a very high mitotic grade. When the patients were age-matched, the tendency toward high mitotic grade persisted (16/27 for HBC *vs* 10/27 for SBC), although the result in this small sample is not formally significant ($p < 0.18$).

Endocrine characteristics

Our case control study of 30 premenopausal white women at 50% risk from HBC-prone families compared with 30 matched SBC controls, showed that: (a) plasma androsterone sulfate was significantly lower in the HBC-risk patients; (b) urinary estrone and estradiol glucuronide, but not estriol glucuronide, were significantly lower; and (c) estrogen conjugation occurred specifically in the post-ovulatory period of the menstrual cycle [32].

Evidence of retrovirus

Detection of reverse transcriptase in a cell population is strong evidence for the presence of a retrovirus, which in humans may be associated with carcinogenesis. Reverse transcriptase activity has recently been reported in cultured peripheral blood monocytes from patients with breast cancer, but not in control patients without cancer [33]. The report is preliminary and has not been verified, but since a retroviral etiology for breast cancer is known in mice and has been suggested in humans, it is of particular interest. If a retroviral etiology should be established for breast cancer, a vertical transmission would be suspected in the cases of FBC and HBC. To account for SBC, horizontal transmission also would need to be postulated. The report is preliminary and needs further investigation.

Oncogene characteristics

An excess of rare alleles of the highly polymorphic c–Harvey–ras–1 oncogene has been reported in breast cancer patient germline DNA as compared to normal controls [34]. In collaboration with the laboratory of Tumor Immunology and Biology at the National Cancer Institute, we have examined this and other polymorphic oncogenic loci in HBC families (cancer-affected and unaffected members) and in normals [35]. We have found no differences in rare allele frequencies between affected and unaffected members of HBC families, although we can find differences when mals [35]. We have found no differences in rare allele frequencies between affected and unaffected members of HBC families, although we can find differences when our pooled set of HBC cases is compared to published gene frequencies. In general, numbers of patients studied so far are too small to draw firm conclusions. If an HBC defect lay on chromosome 11 (the site of these loci) and if germline deletion of genetic materials on one of the homologues is involved in the mechanism of carcinogenesis, we might expect to see a diminution of heterozygosity in the germline DNAs of HBC-prone patients. No such reductions have been observed.

Chromosomal characteristics

Sandberg [36] reported that in the majority of primary and metastatic breast cancers, the karyotype was extremely abnormal and most breast cancer were aneuploid with markers. Trent [37] has found that the chromosomes most commonly altered in breast cancers were 1, 6, 7 and 11. Interestingly, some of these chromosomes are the sites of various c-onc sequences. C-Blym-1, c-N-ras, and c-sk have been mapped to chromosome 1; c-myb to chromosome 6; c-erb-B to chromosome 7; and c-H-ras and c-ets to chromosome 11. Ferti-Passantonopoulou and Panini [38] studying five patients by G banding on direct tumor preparations, have found, in decreasing order of frequency, alterations in chromosomes 1, 3, 5, 6, 11 and 17. In all of the cases, abnormalities of chromosome 1 and 11 were observed. In four of the patients, abnormalities of chromosome 11 showed non-random involvement of q22-23. These investigators concluded that 'band 11q22-23, which has been reported to be an inheritable fragile site and is a specific breakpoint in acute leukemia, may also be specific in a group of breast cancer. Thus, correlation of an inheritable fragile site in a malignant disease with familial incidence seems possible.'

Study of a variety of chromosomal markers of specific tumors has shown that while most are acquired somatically by the tumor, a certain fraction are know to be *constitutional*, such as the 11p13 deletion of Wilms' tumor and the 13q14 deletion in hereditary retinoblastoma. The subsequent deletion of the normal allele may then unmask an otherwise recessive cancer allele. Lundberg *et al.* [39] described tumor *loss of heterozygosity* occurring specifically and non-randomly on chromosome 13 in a small number of cases of ductal carcinoma. These data indicated the possibility that, in these cases, pathogenesis involved a somatic deletion of genetic material which unmasked a recessive breast cancer predisposing allele. In a preliminary study involving HBC families, we have observed an excess of hyperdiploidy in cultured skin fibroblasts, a result that needs further investigation [20].

Educational Programs in HBC

Any cancer control program must provide a clear understanding to the public as to their individual cancer risk, the natural history of hereditary cancer and how these are integrated into a program of surveillance and management [40]. Since the surveillance measures in hereditary breast cancer may differ significantly from recommendations for the general population (because they are specifically adapted to its natural history) the patient and her family physician must clearly understand the rationale behind them.

We initiate an educational program for women at risk for HBC during the midteen years. Each case is handled individually, based upon the intellectual and emotional maturity of the particular adolescent female. Thus, the physician may need to meet on a one-to-one private basis in some circumstances or, in others, it may be preferable to meet with the nuclear family; namely, the patient, her parents, and possibly even one or more of her sisters. The important thing is to try to obtain objectivity for the patient so that she does not single herself out as an object of curiosity, but rather, views her risk status as serious but nevertheless, a concern which can foster positive cancer control results through the earliest possible detection of cancer, should it one day affect her.

During the initial educational session, the pedigree is constructed for the patient, she is identified within its context, and she is permitted an opportunity to ask questions as to the manner in which cancer has occurred throughout her family. Details of the natural history of HBC are then covered. All facets of the surveillance and management program are discussed in depth. The patient is then taught self-breast examination (SBE). She is shown pictures of mammography equipment as well as actual mammograms so that she can better appreciate the significance of this screening measure.

The physician must provide an empathetic listening ear and identify himself as an ally with a strong support role. Because of the emotional crises which some women may experience, it is often necessary to provide a free-wheeling, non-directive, psychotherapeutic setting enabling the patient to discuss her fears and anxieties. Several sessions may be required. The patient then begins formal screening by physician examination during the late-teen years. Each of these sessions should be designed not only for careful examination of the breasts (and other targeted organs should they be accessible for screening and integral to the HBC syndrome of concern) but should also provide reinforcement of all the educational measures discussed above. These follow up sessions should also provide an opportunity for the patient to discuss further her underlying emotional concerns.

Surveillance recommendations

Regular mammography is recommended for all women in their 40s, but is not generally recommended for women in their 20s. These recommendations are mainly based on age-specific risks of breast cancer. It is not considered cost-effective to screen all young women in order to diagnose a few presymptomatically. However, it is possible to identify subgroups of young women at especially high risk for early onset breast cancer, wherein the predictable diagnosic yield will be high and cost effective. One way to target surveillance towards the high risk group is to ask women at risk for HBC to begin mammography at age 25, but in HBC families which include cases diagnosed prior to age 30, high risk females should be under full surveillance at an age which is five years less than the earliest case history in the family. (In an HBC family with multiple early cases, if the youngest diagnosis occurred at age 25, then women at 50% risk from HBC should begin mammography at age 20.) Education and instruction in SBE should begin by their mid-teens.

Eddy *et al.* [41] provide evidence that healthy asymptomatic women between ages 40 and 49 do not show sufficient health or economic benefit from mammography to offset the costs and risks. They contend that the costs for screening this cohort are high and relatively few lives would be saved. Their data indicate that mammography screening in that decade would carry a risk of radiation-induced cancer of the breast of about 1 in 25 000 and conclude that a more prudent approach is to initiate mammography at age 50. The matter of hereditary breast cancer was totally ignored in these reports. HBC family members are clearly one component of a group of women who are at much higher risk for breast cancer prior to age 50 than is the average 'healthy asymptomatic' woman. In this group of women, we believe that the health and economic benefits of mammography far outweigh the costs and risks.

Current state-of-the-art mammography results in a mean glandular dose for a two-view film screen mammogram from 0.05 to 0.15 rads [42]. Despite this low level exposure, concerns still exist over repeated exposure from multiple screening ex aminations. It is known that subtherapeutic radiation dosage ranging from 100 to 2000 rads, can result in a significant excess of breast cancer. Below 100 rads exposure, there is no concrete evidence for an excess of breast cancer occurring. A linear model has been applied to estimate low-dose risk for induction of breast cancer. This linear model represents the upper limits of such risks. Using this estimate, there would be 6.6 excess cancers/10^6 women/year/rad for women exposed at age 40 [43]. Using this figure and applying an average film screen mammography dose of 0.1 rad per breast for a women exposed to yearly mammography from age 20 to age 70, the relative risk for induction of breast cancer for 50 years of screening mammograms would be:

$$6.6 \text{ excess cancers}/10^6 \text{ women/year/rad} \times 50 \text{ years} \times 0.1 \text{ rad} = 33 \text{ excess cancers}/10^6 \text{ women} \times 100 = 0.0033\%$$

Thus, there would be a 0.0033% increased lifetime risk for excess breast cancer from early onset of screening mammography. In a population which faces a 50% risk for hereditary breast cancer, the slightly increased risk of 0.0033% for yearly mammography is negligible.

Surgical implications

Among cases at risk for HBC, those individuals who show poor compliance have breasts that are difficult to examine because of their large size, the presence of marked nodularity due to underlying so-called 'fibrocystic breast disease', the presence of multiple biopsies, marked density of breast tissue with evidence of mammographic dysplasia, and severe cancer phobia, may be candidates for bilateral prophylactic mastectomy. Even stronger candidates for prophylactic mastectomy would be women who have developed unilateral breast cancer, are in the HBC category, and who have early stage disease with likelihood of excellent survival [13].

There are three surgical treatments available to any patient who develops breast cancer, whether they are a member of an HBC family or not. These include: (a) total mastectomy with axillary node dissection (modified radical mastectomy); (b) total mastectomy with axillary node dissection and breast reconstruction; and (c) partial mastectomy with axillary node dissection and whole-breast irradiation [44]. The first two forms of treatment are of equal value and both are employed regularly for the treatment of HBC patients. However, partial mastectomy with axillary node dissection and radiation therapy, although an alternative for patients with sporadic breast cancer, is not recommended in patients with HBC. These patients tend to be much younger and lifetime surveillance (30–50 years) is difficult. The long-term effects of radiation to the affected breast, the contralateral breast, and perhaps more importantly, the surrounding organs, such as the lung and thyroid, are of concern. Nevertheless, this option is occasionally employed if a women expresses a strong desire for breast preservation and is willing to accept the possibility of long-term deleterious effects.

Recommendations for prophylactic surgery to prevent cancer of the breast are based upon highly selective criteria. The first step is to establish clearly the fact that the patient is actually a member of an HBC family. Once their HBC status is confirmed, such high risk women are apprised that because of the autosomal dominant inheritance pattern of this condition, they are at an approximate 50% risk for ultimately developing breast cancer, but that they also have a 50% risk of not developing HBC. We find that the majority of our patients who realize that they also have a 50% chance of *not* developing breast cancer opt for intensive follow-up.

There is a subset of patients, however, in whom prophylactic bilateral mastectomy is felt to be the best course of action. An example would be a patient from an HBC family whose mother and whose daughter have developed breast cancer. It is likely that both the mother and daughter harbor the deleterious gene. The woman who is situated between the two in the genetic line must also carry the gene and is therefore referred to as an obligate gene carrier. Her risk for the development of breast cancer approaches 100%.In addition, recommendation for prophylactic contralateral mastectomy, especially in younger patients, is frequently made due to the inordinately high risk of developing cancer in the opposite breast [45].

When prophylactic mastectomy is recommended, we prefer total mastectomy as opposed to subcutaneous mastectomy. Increasing numbers of reports are appearing in the literature dealing with patients who have developed breast cancer after sucutaneous mastectomy, and it is becoming clear that a significant amount of breast tissue remains after the procedure [46]. These facts, coupled with reconstruction after total mastectomy, make us feel that subcutaneous mastectomy is a procedure which should rarely, if ever, be employed.

Conclusion

About 9% of all breast cancer patients in the United States fit the criteria for HBC, and this implies that their families are prone to HBC. Such high risk families require surveillance and management programs which reflect HBC's natural history, typically the early age of onset, excess bilaterality and specific tumor associations in certain of its heterogeneous forms. The inability to determine who will and who will not manifest breast cancer among the sisters and daughters of breast cancer patients means that the highest possible priority must be given to the search for biological markers which will show women at risk. Also needed are educational programs for patients and physicians so that the significance of HBC is clearly understood.

Acknowledgements

Support for this effort was provided by the Council for Tobacco Research Inc. USA, Grant # 1297C, and by a grant from the Health Futures Foundation.

References

1. Silverberg, E., Lubera, J.A. (1988). Cancer statistics, 1988. *Cancer J. Clin.*, **38**, 5–22.
2. Lynch, H.T. (1981). *Genetics and Breast Cancer*, Van Nostrand Reinhold, New York.
3. Lynch, H.T., Fain, P.R., Goldgar, D., *et al.* (1981). Familial breast cancer and its recognition in an oncology clinic. *Cancer*, **47**, 2730–2739.
4. Petrakis, N.L., Ernster, V., King, M.-C. (1981). Breast cancer. In Schottenfeld, D.S. and Fraumeni, J.F. Jr, (eds.), *Cancer Epidemiology and Prevention*, Saunders, Philadelphia, 855–870.

5. Sattin, R.W., Rubin, G.L., Webster, L.A. *et al.* (1985). Family history and the risk of breast cancer. *J. Amer. Med. Assoc.*, **253**, 1908–1913.
6. Ottman, R., Pike, M.C., King, M.-C., Casagrande, J.T., Henderson, B.E. (1986). Familial breast cancer in a population-based series. *Amer. J. Epidem.*, **123**, 15–21.
7. Go, R.C.P., King, M.-C., Bailey-Wilson, J., Elston, R.C., Lynch, H.T. (1983). Genetic epidemiology of breast and associated cancers in high risk families, Part I. *J. Nat. Cancer Inst.*, **71** 455–462.
8. Lynch, H.T., Krush, A.H., Lemon, H.M. *et al.* (1972). Tumor variation in families with breast cancer. *J. Amer. Med. Ass.*, **222**, 1631–1635.
9. Lynch, H.T., Harris, R.E., Organ, C.H. *et al.* (1978). Familial association of breast/ovarian cancer. *Cancer*, **41**, 1543–1548.
10. Lynch, H.T., Krush, A.J., Guirgis, H. (1973). Genetic factors in families with combined gastrointestinal and breast cancer. *Amer. J. Gastroent.*, **59**, 31–40.
11. Lynch, H.T., Guirgis, H., Brodkey, F. *et al.* (1976). Early age of onset in familial breast cancer. *Arch. Surg.*, **111**, 126–131.
12. Haagensen, C.D., Haagensen, D.E. Jr, Bodian, C. (1981). *Risk and Detection of Breast Cancer*, Saunders, Philadelphia, 10–13.
13. Harris, R.E., Lynch, H.T., Guirgis, H.A. (1978). Familial breast cancer: risk to the contralateral breast. *J. Nat. Cancer Inst.*, **60**,, 955-960.
14. Lynch, H.T., Albano, W.A., Layton, M.A., Kimberling, W.J., Lynch, J.F. (1984). Breast cancer, genetics, and age at first pregnancy. *J. Med. Genet.* **21**, 96–98.
15. Lynch, H.T., Watson, P., Conway, T., Fitzsimmons, M.L., Lynch, J.F. (in press), (1988). Breast cancer family history as a risk factor for early onset breast cancer. *Brit. Cancer Res. Treat.*
16. Lynch, H.T., Mulcahy, G.M., Harris, R.E. *et al.* (1978). Genetic and pathologic findings in a kindred with hereditary sarcoma, breast cancer, brain tumors, leukemia, lung, laryngeal, and adrenal cortical carcinoma. *Cancer*, **41**, 2055–2064.
17. Lynch, H.T., Katz, D.A., Bogard, P.J., Lynch, J.F. (1985). The sarcoma, breast cancer, lung cancer, and adrenocortical carcinoma syndrome revisited; childhood cancer. *Amer J. Dis. Child.*, **139**, 134–136.
18. King, M.-C., Go, R.C.P., Bailey-Wilson, ??. *et al.* (1983). Genetic epidemiology of breast and associated cancers in high risk families, Part II. *J. Nat. Cancer Inst.*, **71**, 463.
19. Albano, W.A., Recabaren, J.A., Lynch, H.T. *et al.* (1982). Natural history of hereditary cancer of the breast and colon. *Cancer*, **50**, 360–363.
20. Lynch, H.T., Albano, W.A., Danes, B.S. *et al.* (1984). Genetic predisposition to breast cancer. *Cancer*, **53**, 612–622.
21. Lynch, H.T., Lynch, J.F. (1986). Breast cancer genetics in an oncology clinic: 328 consecutive patients. *Ca. Genet. Cytogenet.*, **22**, 369.371.
22. DuPont, W.D., Page, D.L. (1985). Risk factors for breast cancer in women with proliferative breast disease. *N. Engl. J. Med.*, **312**, 146–151.
23. DuPont, W.D., Page, D.L. (1987). Breast cancer risk associated with proliferative disease, age at first birth, and a family history of breast cancer. *Amer. J. Epidem.*, **125**, 769–779.
24. Page, D.L., DuPont, W.D., Rogers, L.W., Rados, M.S. (1985). Atypical hyperplastic lesions of the female breast: a long term followup study. *Cancer*, **55**, 2698–2708.
25. Rosen, P.P., Holmes, G., Lesser, M.L., Kinne, D.W., Beattie, E.J. (1985). Juvenile papillomatosis and breast carcinoma. *Cancer*, **55**, 1345–1352.
26. Lagios, M.D., Rose, M.R., Margolin, F.R. (1980). Tubular carcinoma of the breast: association with multicentricity, bilaterality, and family history of mammary carcinoma. *Amer. J. Clin. Path.*, **23**, 25–30.
27. Anderson, D.E. (1974). Genetic study of breast cancer: identification of a high risk group. *Cancer*, **34**, 1090–1097.

28. Rosen, P.P., Lesser, M.L., Senie, R.T., Kinne, D.W. (1982). Epidemiology of breast carcinoma, III. A clinicopathologic study with a 10 year followup. *Cancer*, **50**, 171–179.
29. Mulcahy, G.M., Platt, R. (1982). Pathologic aspects of familial carcinoma of the breast. In H.T. Lynch (ed.), *Genetics and Breast Cancer*, Van Nostrand Reinhold, New York, 65.
30. Marcus, J., Page, D., Watson, P., Conway, T., Lynch, XX (1988). High mitotic grade in hereditary breast cancer. *Lab. Invest.*, **58**, 61A.
31. Ridolfi, R.L., Rosen, P.P., Port, A. *et al.* (1977). Medullary carcinoma of the breast. *Cancer*, **40**, 1365–1385.
32. Fishman, J., Bradlow, H.L., Fukushima, D. *et al.* (1983). Abnormal estrogen conjugation in women at risk for familial breast cancer is concentrated at the periovulatory stage of the menstrual cycle. *Cancer. Res.*, **43**, 1884–1890.
33. Al-Sumidaie, A.M., Leinster, S.J., Hart, C.A., Green, C.D., McCarthy, K. (1988). Particles with properties of retrovirus in monocytes from patients with breast cancer. *Lancet*, **i**, 5–8.
34. Lidereau, R., Escot, C., Theillet, C., *et al.* (1986). High frequency of rare alleles of the human c-Ha-*ras*-1 proto-oncogene in breast cancer patients. *J. Nat. Cancer Inst.*, **77**, 697–701.
35. Lynch, H.T., Watson, P., Marcus, J.N. *et al.* (1987). Hereditary breast cancer: search for biomarkers. *J. Tum. Mark. Onc.*, **2**, 153.159.
36. Sandberg, A.A. (1980). *The Chromosomes in Human Cancer and Leukemia*, Elsevier, New York, 485.
37. Trent, J.M. (1985). Cytogenetic and molecular biologic alterations in human breast cancer: a review. *Brit. Cancer Res. Treat.*, **5**, 221.229.
38. Ferti-Passantonopoulou, A.D., Panini, A.D. (1987). Common cytogenetic findings in primary breast cancer. *Ca. Genet. Cytogenet.*, **27**, 289–298.
39. Lundberg, C., Skoog, L., Cavenee, W.K., Nordenskjold, M. (1987). Loss of heterozygosity in human ductal breast tumors indicates a recessive mutation on choromosome 11. *Proc. Nat. Acad. Sci., Wash*, **84**, 2372–2376.
40. Lynch, H.T., Conway, T., Watson, P., Schreiman, J., Fitzgibbons, R.J. Jr (1988). Extremely early onset hereditary breat cancer (HBC): surveillance/management implications. *Neb. Med. J.*, **73**, 97–100.
41. Eddy, D., Hasselblad, V., McGivney, W., Hendee, W. (1988). The value of mammography screening in women under age 50 years. *J. Amer. Med. Ass.*, **259**, 1512–1519.
42. Committee of the Biological Effects of Ionizing Radiations (1980). *The Effects on Populations of Exposure to Low Levels of Ionizing Radiation: 1980)*, National Academy Press, 269–285.
43. Holland, R., Hendricks, J.H.C., Mravunac, M. (1983). Mammographically occult breast cancer. *Cancer*, **52**, 1810–1819.
44. Fitzgibbons, R.J. Jr., Anthone, G. (1987). Changing concepts in the surgical treatment of patients with curable breast cancer. In Lynch, H.T., Kullander, S. (eds.), *Cancer Genetics in Women*, CRC Press, Boca Raton.
45. Lynch, H.T., Conway, T., Fitzgibbons, R.J. Jr. *et al.* Age of onset heterogeneity in hereditary breast cancer, Parts I and II. Submitted to *Brit. Cancer Res. Treat.*
46. Goodnight, J.E. Jr, Quagliana, J.M., Morton, D.L. (1984). Failure of subcutaneous mastectomy to prevent the development of breast cancer. *J. Surg. Onc.*, **26**, 198–201.

Chapter 4

Hormonal and Reproductive Factors – New Evidence

M. JAWED IQBAL and W. TAYLOR

Introduction

Three major hormone-related events in the life of a women influence the risk of her developing breast cancer. These events are: age at onset of menstruation (menarche), age at the menopause, and age at which she has her first full-term pregnancy (FFTP). In Western women, breast cancer risk is *increased* by an early menarche, a late menopause, or a late FFTP.

The risk for breast cancer associated with early menarche is particularly important in cancers developing in the younger age group; in women whose menarche occurs before the age of 12 years the risk is twice that of those who experience menarche after the age of 13 years [1]. Women who have a natural menopause before reaching the age of 45 years are only half as much at risk as those whose menopause occurs after the age of 55; this lowered risk applies also when an artificial menopause is induced by elimination of ovarian function [2]. Women who have a FFTP before the age of 20 years are exposed to only half the risk of that of childless women. However, childless women are not as much at risk as those whose FFTP occurs after the age of 35 [3].

Those relationships indicate that the hormonal status of a woman has a profound influence on her susceptibility to breast cancer, and therefore numerous studies have attempted to define the hormone secretion patterns which might indicate that a particular woman is a more likely candidate for breast cancer. The results of these case-controlled studies have proved to be confusing, and investigations are now made more complicated by the introduction of hormonal agents which profoundly affect the normal endocrine function of women. The most important of those agents are the steroidal oral contraceptives, and the hormonal preparations which are used to ameliorate the symptoms of the menopause (i.e., hormone replacement therapy).

Role of Oestrogens

There is no doubt that the sex hormonal steroids, particularly the oestrogens, are implicated in the aetiology of breast cancer. However, it is now believed that sex steroids act mainly as promoters rather than as initiators of carcinogenesis, i.e., they do not induce the initial events of carcinogenesis, but rather they are involved in the processes which lead to the progression of lesions which have been rendered potentially malignant by agents or factors other than the steroids themselves. The traditional suspicion about the role of oestrogens as carcinogens probably emanates from earlier experiments with the powerful non-steroidal, synthetic compound diethylstilboestrol (DES) which undoubtedly has carcinogenic potential. DES and related compounds are now very little used in human therapeutics.

The main criticisms of clinical studies which have concentrated on the role of oestrogens in breast cancer are as follows:

(i) Over the past decade evidence has accumulated which suggests that sex steroids such as oestrogens, androgens and progestins act in concert. Although many of the actions of oestrogens and androgens are mutually antagonistic, examples of synergistic action do exist. The actions of progestins are closely interlinked with those of oestrogens in bringing about a response in target organs. However, most natural and synthetic progestins, particularly those used in contraceptives, have some androgenic activity enabling them to act as androgen agonists or antagonists [reviewed in 4, 5]. Thus, in studies of the role of oestrogens in breast cancer the action of androgens and progestins must be taken into account.

(ii) Sex hormone binding globulin (SHBG) has been studied either in the calculation of biologically active free oestradiol [reviewed in 4, 5] or in relation to established breast cancer risk factors [6]. However, the conclusions even of these studies are open to doubt because of misunderstanding about the roles of SHBG and serum albumin. Most studies have emphasised the role of SHBG in regulating the ratio of biologically active androgens, implying that it is that ratio, and not the total amounts of either hormone group, which determines the overall oestrogenic or androgenic effect. In fact, SHBG binds the most biologically potent androgen dihydrotestosterone (DHT) with an affinity three times greater than that of oestradiol; and testosterone, the precursor of DHT, has an affinity for SHBG which is nearly double that of oestradiol. Therefore, for any given increase in the amounts of SHBG there will be proportionally greater amounts of oestradiol than of androgens available for biological action. This has led to the concept of SHBG being an 'oestrogen amplifier' [7, 8].

Role of Early Menarche

With the reservations expressed above, hormonal secretion pattern data lend support to observations in case-control studies of this being a high risk group, and also tend to confirm the findings of epidemiological studies [1]. Higher oestradiol levels are found in the serum of girls with early menarche, and are associated with early establishment of ovulatory cycles [9]. In these girls, the higher the concentrations of oestradiol found in the follicular phase, the greater was the likelihood that the cycle would be ovulatory, whereas the reverse applied to testosterone levels. The relatively higher oestradiol levels also persisted at ages when the differences in the frequency of ovulatory cycles were disappearing, suggesting that women in the high risk group have higher production of oestradiol than women with a lower risk. It was also found that the women with early menarche with ovulatory cycles had a higher Quetelet Index of adiposity (weight/height).

Two other hormonal factors may be involved in the risk associated with early ovulatory cycles. One is an increase in serum prolactin levels [10], and the other is a variation in testosterone secretion during the menstrual cycle [10]. This latter observation underlines the importance of the oestrogen:androgen balance and the importance of SHBG as a determinant of that ratio [7, 8].

Role of Pregnancy

As mentioned above, an early FFTP is thought to reduce the risk of breast cancer [3, 6, 11]. Those who postulate that oestradiol is indeed a carcinogen suggest that the reduction in bioavailable oestrogen (due to the elevated SHBG levels found in pregnancy) is the reason why early pregnancy protects women against breast cancer [6, 11]. Recent evidence, however, demonstrates that there is a decrease in serum prolactin levels after the FFTP, suggesting that other hormonal factors may be involved. Again, little attention has been paid to the proportionate increase in free oestradiol in relation to androgens, although the levels of androgens and oestrogens are both greatly elevated during pregnancy [12].

It seems that an early FFTP, around the age of 20 years, reduces breast cancer risk by half compared with childless women, who definitely constitute a high risk group [6, 11]. It is possible that the protective effect of a pregnancy may result from the alteration in the physiology of the breast or the responsiveness of breast tissue to the carcinogenic effect of hormones.

Role of Early Menopause

Many studies have shown that an early menopause reduces the risk of breast cancer [2, 6, 11]. In the literature the terms 'menopause' and 'climacteric' are often used synonymously, but a correct definition of such terms is important because hormonal patterns differ during the months leading to, during or after the menopause. The 'climacteric' may be defined as an event in the reproductive life of a woman when she changes sexually and physically as she approaches old age. A period of at least six months after cessation of menses should be allowed to elapse before a women is considered as postmenopausal [6, 11].

With the onset of the menopause, serum levels of prolactin, sex steroids of ovarian origin (oestrogens and androgens) and of SHBG decrease [6, 11]. These changes may reflect the balance of the oestrogen:androgen ratio which appears to be lower in the early postmenopausal years [12, 13]. Thus, the woman with an early menopause is protected from the possible harmful effects of free oestrogens.

Obesity and the Role of Androgens

The observation that obese postmenopausal women have an increased risk of breast cancer (see Chapter 6) is usually ascribed to the increased conversion of androgens to oestrogens by the aromatase system because such conversion is known to occur in adipose tissue [11]. In addition, obese women tend to have lower levels of SHBG because of the hormone imbalance resulting from the conversions described above, and also because of interconversions of sex hormones in other peripheral tissues. Before the menopause, the inverse relationship between SHBG and body weight it not as pronounced as it is after the menopause, and for a given body weight the SHBG decreases less in premenopausal than in postmenopausal women [6].

Several reports have implicated androgens as aetiological factors in breast cancer in women [reviewed in 4, 5], and comparison of enzyme activities in normal and cancerous breast tissue also indicates that androgens might stimulate breast cancer growth [14]. An accumulation of intracellular SHBG has been found in breast cancer but not in normal breast tissue [5], and it has been suggested that this intracellular SHBG acts to concentrate the sex steroids locally in malignant breast tissue. In the case of male breast cancer, the potent antiandrogen cyproterone acetate is an effective agent in treatment [15].

Racial Differences in Breast Cancer Incidence

The relatively low incidence of breast cancer amongst Japanese women is well documented (see Chapter 2). It may be partly explained by the recent discovery of a new, specific sex steroid binding protein, fetal steroid binding protein (FSBP), which behaves very much like SHBG when in a purified or partially purified form [4, 5]. The serum levels of the protein were compared in two populations; a 'low risk' group consisting of 56 Japanese women (45 premenopausal) and a 'high risk' group of 59 British women (25 premenopausal). Higher levels of FSBP were found in the Japanese women overall, and the premenopausal Japanese women had relatively higher levels than the premenopausal British women. Also, there was a significant negative correlation with age in both populations, the correlation being much higher in the postmenopausal women. The interaction of FSBP with other steroid binding proteins has a bearing on the amount of biologically available sex steroids.

Conclusion

In spite of the widespread use of oral contraceptives and hormonal replacement therapy in Western populations, there is no unequivocal evidence that these agents increase the overall risk of breast cancer (see Chapter 8). However, within the population there is a need to assess the possible risk for a particular woman or small groups of women. For instance, in the United Kingdom very young women, some even under 16 years of age, are being prescribed oral contraceptives apparently without regard to the age of menarche and subsequent duration of use. Such long-term users may be at risk, particularly if they postpone their first pregnancy to an age when the risk of breast cancer becomes significantly increased. Again, the menopause can begin as early as 35 years, and the use of oral contraceptives and/or hormone replacement therapy may delay the natural menopause and hence increase the risk of breast cancer appearing subsequently.

It will become increasingly important for the physician to consider each individual women on the basis of the overall risks and benefits arising from the use of such hormonal agents, and also to be aware of the factors contributing to such risks. Nevertheless, the reproductive life of the woman and her steroid hormone secretions and intake are only a part of a complex sequence of events which might lead to breast cancer.

References

1. Pike, M., Henderson, B.E., Casagrande, J.T., Rosario, I., Gray, G.E. (1981). Oral contraceptive use and early abortion as risk factors for beast cancer in young women. *Brit. J. Cancer*, **43**, 72–76
2. Trichopoulos, D., MacMahon, B., Cole, P. (1972). Menopause and breast cancer risk. *J. Nat. Cancer Inst.*, **48**, 605–613.
3. MacMahon, B., Cole, P., Lin, T.M., *et al.* (1970). Age at first birth and breast cancer risk. *Bull. World Hlth. Org.*, **43**, 209.217.
4. Iqbal, M.J. (1986, 1987). Sex-steroid binding proteins and breast disease – a view. *Breast News International*, Part I. **2**, 8–10; Part II, **2**, 7–8.
5. Iqbal, M.J., Colletta, A.A., Valyani, S.H. (1987). Sex-steroid receptors and cancer – are we back on the right tracks? Review, *Anticancer Res.*, **7**, 773–780.
6. Moore, J.W., Key, T.J.A., Bulbrook, R.D., Clark, C.M.G., Allen, D.S., Wang, D.Y., Pike, M.C. (1987). Sex hormone binding globulin and risk factors for breast cancer in a population of normal women who had never used exogenous sex hormones. *Brit. J. Cancer*, **56**, 661–666.
7. Anderson, D.C. (1974). Sex hormone binding globulin. *Clin. Endocrinol.*, **3**, 69–96.
8. Englebienne, P. (1984). The serum steroid proteins. In *Molec. Aspects Med.*, Vol. 7, Pergamon Press, London, 313–396.
9. Vihko, R., Apter, D. (1984). Endocrine characteristics of adolescent menstrual cycles: impact of early menarche. *J. Steroid Biochem.*, **20**, 231–236.
10. L'Hermite, M. (1976). Prolactin. In Loraine, J.A. and Bell, E.T. (eds.), *Hormone Assays and Their Clinical Applications*, 4th edn. Churchill Livingstone, New York, 293–322.
11. Pike, M.C., Krailo, M.D., Henderson, B.E., Casagrande, J.T., Hoel, D.G. (1983). Hormonal risk factors, breast tissue age and the age-incidence of breast cancer. *Nature*, **303**, 767–770.
12. Vermeulen, A. (1979). The androgens: In *Hormones in Blood*, 3rd edn. Gray, C.H., James, V.H.T. (eds.), vol. 3, Academic Press, New York, 354–416.
13. Jaszmann, L.J.B. (1976). Epidemiology of the climacteric syndrome. In Campbell, S. (ed.), *The Management of the Menopause and Postmenopausal Years*, MTP Press, Lancaster, 2–23.
14. Vermeulen, A., Deslypere, J.P., Paridaens, R. (1986). Steroid dynamics in the normal and carcinomatous mammary gland. *J. Steroid Biochem.*, **25**, 799–802.
15. Lopez, M. (1985). Cyproterone acetate in the treatment of metastatic cancer of the male breast. *Cancer*, **55**, 2334–2336.

Chapter 5

Relationship to Previous Breast Disease

WILLIAM D. DUPONT and DAVID L. PAGE

Introduction

It has been known for several decades that women with benign breast lesions are at increased risk of breast cancer. Numerous studies have shown that women who have undergone biopsies for benign breast lesions have a breast cancer risk higher than that of the general population although its estimated magnitude ranges from 1.5 to 4.8 in different studies [1, 2]. This risk has caused great concern among women, particularly in view of the high prevalence of painful, lumpy breasts in women approaching the menopause. It has led to ever-increasing numbers of patients undergoing breast biopsy for diagnosis, particularly in the United States.

Benign breast lesions have a highly variable microscopic appearance ranging from normal breast tissue through to carcinoma *in situ*. Thus, fibroadenoma, sclerosing adenosis and papilloma each has a distinctive appearance and is associated with a different age distribution, so that there is no reason to consider all women who have undergone benign breast biopsies as having the same disease. Another problem is that it is not always easy to distinguish between pathologic and physiologic changes. Indeed, in view of the increasing frequency of histologic evaluation of breasts, and the rarity of a diagnosis of 'normal breast tissue' it is likely that many women with 'biopsy confirmed benign breast disease' have histologically normal breasts.

This chapter will categorize the microscopic changes seen in benign breast lesions into diagnostic groups. It will also discuss the cancer risks associated with these diagnoses and how these risks may be multiplied in the presence of other recognisable risk factors in the patient.

The Microscopic Spectrum of Benign Breast Disease

The borderline between invasive cancer and benign breast disease is *in situ* carcinoma, which has all of the anatomic characteristics of malignancy except the ability to invade surrounding tissue. The characteristics of *in situ* carcinoma are extreme levels of cellular proliferation, cytologic atypia, and histologic atypia; in other words, excessive numbers of highly abnormal cells grouped together in highly unusual patterns. Benign lesions occupy the broad continuum between normal tissue and *in situ* carcinoma and vary both in their degree of hyperplasia and their degree of atypia. Thus, lesions with florid hyperplasia but no sign of atypia are common, while lesions with marked atypia but mild hyperplasia, although rare, are also found.

Table 5.1 Risk estimates for invasive carcinoma approved by the College of American Pathologists (adapted from Hutter *et al.* [6])

No increased risk (Non-proliferative disease)
Adenosis, either sclerosing or florid [1]
Duct estasia
Mild epithelial hyperplasia of usual type
Slightly increased risk (1.5–2 times) (Epithelial proliferative disease without atypia)
Hyperplasia of usual type, moderate or florid
Moderately increased risk (4–5 times) (Atypical hyperplasia)[2]
Atypical ductal hyperplasia
Atypical lobular hyperplasia
High risk (8–10 times) (Carcinoma *in situ*)
Lobular carcinoma *in situ*
Ductal carcinoma *in situ* (smaller and microscopic examples of non-comedo DCIS)

[1] This lesion rests in the 'no elevation of risk' category despite the presentation by Dupont and Page [2] of sclerosing adenosis in the slightly in creased risk category. Sclerosing adenosis had not been previously found to be associated with elevated risk, however McDivitt *et al.* have recently reported a slight elevation of cancer risk for these lesions (1988; *Lab. Invest.*, **58**, 62A).
[2] The atypical hyperplastic lesions differ somewhat in age incidence and interval to appearance of later cancer [13] but are associated with the same magnitude of risk elevation.

Several authors have proposed histologic classification schemes for breast lesions [3–5] and all these systems are closely related. Our own system (Table 1) which draws heavily from the other two has been endorsed by the College of American Pathologists [6] and can be summarized as follows. First, all benign breast tissue is classified as having or lacking proliferative disease. Proliferative disease indicates increased cancer risk and is characterized by at least moderate epithelial hyperplasia. These lesions often have five or more cells above the basement membrane and tend to cross and distend spaces. They are commonly recognized as 'papillomatosis' or 'epitheliosis' without atypia. Non-proliferative tissue may be either normal or may contain lesions such as cysts, calcifications or mild hyperplasias. Mild hyperplasias have three of four cells above the basement membrane, rather than the normal complement of two. They also have little tendency to cross over or distend spaces.

Proliferative lesions are further divided into those that contain atypical hyperplasia and those that do not. Lesions with atypical hyperplasia have some but not all of the characteristics of *in situ* carcinoma. They possess both cytologic and morphologic atypia, but lack the degree of hyperplasia or atypia required for a diagnosis of *in situ* carcinoma. Proliferative lesions that lack atypia (PDWA) include moderate and florid ductal hyperplasias and papillomas. It is important to emphasize that lesions with atypical hyperplasia are relatively rare.

We diagnosed atypia in only 4% of a consecutive series of 10 366 benign lesions [2]. PDWA was diagnosed in 27% of these biopsies while the remainder were found to be non-proliferative. A potential source of confusion is the difference between atypia as used here and the atypia score of Black and Chabon [5]. In the Black and Chabon system, lesions with atypia scores of 3 or 4 are described as atypical. However, when Kodlin *et al.* [7] applied this system to a consecutive cohort of 2403 women, 13% were found to have atypia, suggesting considerably less stringent criteria.

In current series the proportion of biopsies with atypia may differ from that found in our study because today most biopsies result from a suspicious mammogram. Rubin *et al.* [8] found atypical hyperplasia in 10% of biopsies performed for mammographically detected non-palpable lesions while Bartow *et al.* [9] found atypical hyperplasia in 2.5% of a forensic autopsy study of non-Hispanic white women who were at least 40 years of age.

What is the Cancer Risk Associated with Benign Breast Disease?

Several authors have studied the relationship between different types of benign breast disease and the risk of breast cancer [2, 7, 10–14]. In our retrospective cohort study [2] all benign breast biopsies performed at three local hospitals between 1952 and 1968 were re-evaluated using our classification and we then determine the current whereabouts of a sub-cohort of these women. A total of 3300 patients or their next of kin were interviewed, representing 84% of those eligible for follow-up. The median follow-up interval was 17 years. The patient's cancer outcome and other epidemiologic information was obtained at the time of the interview and, if positive, was confirmed. The observed cancer morbidity was then compared to that of women of comparable age and length of follow-up from a suitable reference population.

Table 5.2 Relative risk of breast cancer among women who have undergone breast biopsy revealing benign tissue (Dupont and Page [2])

	Frequency of diagnosis (%)	*Relative risk*[1]	*95% confidence interval*
Atypical hyperplasia (AH)	3.6	4.4	3.1–6.3
Proliferative disease without AH	26.7	1.6	1.3–2.0
Proliferative disease (PD)	30.3	1.9	1.6–2.3
No PD	69.7	0.89	0.62–1.3
All study subjects	100.0	1.5	1.3–1.8

[1] Calculated with respect to women from the Third National Cancer Survey in Atlanta. Adjusted for age at biopsy and length of follow-up.

The major findings of this study are summarized in Table 2. Women with atypical hyperplasia have 4.4 times the invasive breast cancer risk of that of women from the general population of the same age group. Of women undergoing benign biopsies, 70% lack proliferative disease and are not at increased breast cancer risk compared to women of similar age who have not been biopsied. In contrast, atypical hyperplasia was found in only 4% of study subjects but was associated with a substantial increase in breast cancer risk. Kodlin *et al.* [7] studied a cohort of 2400 women who have undergone benign breast biopsy. The women in their study had a substantially higher overall risk of breast cancer than did those in ours (relative risk = 2.5 *vs* 1.5). Their relative risk for grade 4 atypia was 6.0, which is roughly comparable to our diagnosis of atypical hyperplasia after correcting for the overall difference in relative risk between these studies.

Our study suggested that calcification was an important risk factor in women with proliferative disease. Among women with atypical hyperplasia, the presence of calcification raised the relative risk of breast cancer from 4.0 to 6.5. This result is in agreement with Hutchinson *et al.* [11] who found that the presence of calcification in women with epithelial hyperplasia or papillomatosis raised the relative risk of breast cancer from 2.8 to 5.3. The presence of calcification in women without proliferative disease did not raise cancer risk in either study. Cysts in the absence of other risk factors did not elevate breast cancer risk in women from our biopsied cohort. The overall cancer risk for women with cysts is very close to that for all women in the study. This result is in agreement with that reported by Hutchinson *et al.* [11].

Guidelines for *in Situ* Carcinoma

Palpable comedo carcinoma *in situ* is universally accepted as a true cancer; these large lesions have long been recognized as having a high likelihood of developing into invasive cancer. Microscopic examples of carcinoma *in situ*, however, are perhaps best thought of as high risk premalignant neoplasms. In particular, non-comedo forms of microscopic *in situ* ductal carcinoma have been demonstrated to be associated with a risk of invasive carcinoma development in the range of about 25% within 15 years [15]. The relative risk for these patients, controlled for age, is about 10 times that of the general population.

Lobular carcinoma *in situ* might be viewed as a high risk lesion rather than as a carcinoma. Lobular carcinoma *in situ* is associated with a risk of later development of breast carcinoma 8 to 9 times that of the general population controlled for age [16, 17]. The major difference between these types of microscopic carcinoma *in situ* is that lobular carcinoma *in situ* is followed by the development of invasive carcinoma equally in either breast, whereas the later carcinomas developing after microscopic ductal carcinoma *in situ* regularly developed at the site where the previous carcinoma *in situ* was manifest [15].

This background information on carcinoma *in situ* reflects the difficulty in deciding therapy in these cases. Many people currently follow-up women with lobular carcinoma *in situ* with mammography on a regular basis but a decision will be made according to the woman's level of concern, the feasibility of obtaining mammograms, etc. Certainly, non-comedo ductal carcinoma *in situ* lesions of 1–2 cm in size which are technically amenable to excision with a rim of normal tissue can be adequately treated in this fashion. Recurrence are unusual and are usually of *in situ* disease [18, 19]. Whether radiation should then be considered is controversial [20].

Other Factors Multiplying the Breast Cancer Risk

The cancer risk of a women with benign breast disease is affected also by several other established risk factors for breast cancer [21]. We have shown a synergistic (or addictive) effect between some of these factors and proliferative disease, in increasing a woman's breast cancer risk [2, 22].

Table 3 shows the effect of a first degree family history of breast cancer (mother, sister or daughter), on patients from our study cohort. In this table, the relative risks in each subgroup are calculated with respect to a different reference category. For example, the lower half of the table shows the effect of age at first birth and family history on breast cancer risk, and the relative risks in this subgroup are calculated with respect to women without a family history who gave birth by age 20. Women with a family history who gave birth after age 30 are at 5.1 times the risk of women who gave birth by age 20 and have no family history of the disease.

Our observations thus agree with those of MacMahon *et al.* [23] and others [21] concerning the protective effects of early age at first birth on breast cancer risk and this effect is particularly pronounced among women with a family history of breast cancer. Table 3 also shows that there is an important interaction between family history and proliferative disease. Women with both atypia and a family history have a cancer risk that is comparable to that of women with non-comedo ductal carcinoma *in situ* [15].

Table 5.3 Relative risk of breast cancer associated with a family history[1] and other variables in women who have undergone benign breast biopsies (95% confidence intervals are given in parentheses)

	No family history		*Family history*	
All patients	1.0[1]		1.8	(1.2–2.8)
No proliferative disease (No PD)	1.0[2]		1.4	(0.48–3.9)
PD without atypia	1.9	(1.2–3.0)	2.7	(1.4–5.3)
Atypical hyperplasia	4.3	(2.4–7.8)	11.0	(5.5–24)
No cysts	1.0[2]		1.6	(0.55–4.6)
Cysts	1.3	(0.88–2.0)	2.7	(1.5–4.6)
Age at first birth (years)				
≤ 20	1.0[2]		0.64	(0.08–4.8)
21–29	1.5	(0.83–2.8)	2.7	(1.2–6.0)
≥ 30	1.2	(0.51–2.9)	5.1	(1.8–1.4)
Nulliparous	1.7	0.91–3.3)	3.4	(1.4–7.8)

1 Mother, sister or daughter with breast cancer.
2 Reference category (denominator of relative risks in the subgroup).

Several studies have found an increased risk of benign breast disease associated with intake of caffeine [24, 25], and some women report a marked improvement in their symptoms after removing caffeine from their diet. Oral contraceptives are known to be protective against benign breast disease although not against breast cancer development (see Chapter 8). Li Volsi *et al.* [26] found that the pill reduced the frequency of benign lesions with little or no epithelial hyperplasia but not of lesions with marked proliferative disease or atypia. This finding, which has not been confirmed by others, suggests that oral contraceptives may protect against the types of breast disease that are not associated with increased cancer risk.

The effect of age at first birth or nulliparity was more marked among women with proliferative disease. Table 4 shows the effect of proliferative disease, age at first birth, and breast size on cancer risk (breast size being determined by the patients' self evaluation.) Breast size had little effect on cancer risk among women without proliferative disease, but among women with proliferative disease, breast cancer risk increased with increasing breast size. Many authors have found that breast cancer risk is elevated in overweight women [21]. Our results would agree with this finding although breast size was a better predictor of cancer risk than the standard measure of body build (weight/height^2.)

Table 5.4 Relative risk of breast cancer associated with proliferative disease and age at first birth and breast size in women who have undergone benign breast biopsies (95% confidence intervals are given in parentheses)

	No proliferative disease	*Proliferative disease without atypia*	*Atypical hyperplasia*
Age at first birth (years)			
≤ 20	1.0[1]	2.2 (0.61 6.8)	3.6 (0.65–20)
21–29	1.5 (0.47–4.7)	3.0 (1.0–8.5)	10.0 (3.3–31)
≥ 30	1.9 (0.42–8.4)	3.5 (1.0–12)	10.0 (3.3–31)
Nulliparous	2.1 (0.64–6.8)	3.3 (1.1–9.8)	11.0 (3.6–36)
		Proliferative diseases	
Breast size			
Small	1.0[1]	1.8 (0.69–4.4)	
Medium	0.9 (0.35–2.3)	2.1 (0.89–4.9)	
Large	1.2 (0.33–4.1)	3.0 (1.2–7.9)	

[1] Reference category (denominator of relative risks for this subgroup).

In 1976 Wolfe [27] described mammographic parenchymal patterns which he postulated would be associated with increased risk of breast cancer. These patterns are characterized either by (a) severe involvement with a prominent ductal pattern in at least one-fourth of the breast volume (P2), or (b) severe involvement with dysplasia which often obscures the underlying ductal pattern (DY). Many authors have investigated the cancer risk associated with these patterns [28, 29, 30]. Although the findings of some of these studies are inconsistent, it appears that the P2 and DY patterns are associated with a 2- to 5-fold increase in breast cancer risk. The relationship between these patterns and epithelial hyperplasia is unclear, with different authors reporting contradictory results [28]. Bright *et al.* [31] have reported an association between epithelial hyperplasia and extensive nodular densities in post-menopausal women.

Thermography is not utilized as a detection tool for breast cancer because mammography is so much more sensitive and specific in detecting breast cancers. Whether thermography might be useful in indicating women at increased or degreased risk for breast cancer development in certain age groups has not yet been proven. Clinical investigations have failed to reveal a difference in predictive accuracy between the xeromammographic and screen-film techniques for mammography [32]. Serum levels of markers such as selenium are said to be useful as determinants of breast cancer risk, but have not been tested in a prospective manner.

Conclusion

The terms 'fibrocystic disease' and 'benign breast disease' have been applied to a wide spectrum of conditions ranging from cyclically painful or lumpy breasts through to *in situ* carcinoma. The knowledge that, as a group, these women are at increased breast cancer risk has caused great concern, and has, in some instances, resulted in women having their insurance policies cancelled or their premiums raised.

In view of this concern, perhaps the most important finding of the recent research on benign breast disease is that 70% of women undergoing benign breast biopsies are not at increased cancer risk. Although this result was obtained for women who underwent breast biopsy, it is probably safe to conclude that it applies to all women who suffer from breast pain or lumpiness that ebbs and flows with their menstrual cycle. Such women can be reassured that they are not at greater cancer risk than other women of their age, although this knowledge does nothing to relieve the patients' symptoms.

The American Cancer Society recommends annual mammographic screening for all women after age 50 but the costs of such a program make it unlikely that all such women will be regularly screened world-wide. (There is considerable controversy concerning the value of mammography for women before their fifth decade). However, women with proliferative disease in the breast are at increased risk and need to be followed carefully. They should be urged to have regular mammograms and for women with evidence of atypical hyperplasia, annual clinical examinations including mammography are mandatory.

References

1. Ernster, V.L. (1981). The epidemiology of benign breast disease. *Epidemiol. Rev.*, 3, 184–202.
2. Dupont, W.D. and Page, D.L. (1985). Risk factors for breast cancer in women with proliferative breast disease. *N. Engl. J. Med.*, **312**, 146–151.
3. Page, D.L., Anderson, T.J., Rogers, L.W. (1987). Epithelial hyperplasia. In *Diagnostic Histopathology of the Breast*, Churchill Livingstone, Edinburgh, 120–156.
4. Wellings, S.R., Jensen, H.M., Marcum, R.G. (1975). An atlas of subgross pathology of the human breast with special reference to possible precancerous lesions. *J. Nat. Cancer Inst.*, **55**, 231–273.
5. Black, M.M., Chabon, A.B. (1969). *In situ* carcinoma of the breast. In: Sommers, S.C. (ed.), *Pathology Annual*, Appleton-Century-Crofts, New York, 185–210.

6. Hutter, R.V.P. *et al.* (1986). Is 'fibriocystic disease' of the breast precancerous? consensus meeting, 3–5 Oct. 1985, New York; convened by the Cancer Committee of the College of American Pathologists; supported by a grant from the American Cancer Society. *Arch. Path. Lab. Med.*, **110**, 171–173.
7. Kodlin, D., Winger, E.E., Morgenstern, N.L., Chen, U. (1977). Chronic mastopathy and breast cancer: a follow-up study. *Cancer*, **39**, 2603–2607.
8. Rubin, E., Alexander, R.W., Visscher, D.W. *et al.* (1988). Proliferative disease and atypia in biopsies performed for mammographically detected nonpalpable lesions. *Cancer*, in press.
9. Bartow, S.A., Pathak, D.R., Black, W.C. *et al.* (1987). Prevalence of benign, atypical, and malignant breast lesions in populations at different risk for breast cancer. *Cancer*, **60**, 2751–2760.
10. Black, M.M., Barclay, T., Cutler, S.J., Hankey, B.F., Asire, A.J. (1972). Association of atypical characteristics of benign breast leasions with subsequent risk of breast cancer. *Cancer*, **29**, 338–343.
11. Hutchinson, W.B., Thomas, D.B., Hamlin, W.B., Roth, G.J., Peterson, A.V., Williams, B. (1980). Risk of breast cancer in women with benign breast disease. *J. Nat. Cancer Inst.*, **65**, 13–20.
12. Haagensen, C.D., Bodian, C., Haagensen, D.E. Jr (1981). *Breast Cancer Risk and Detection*, Saunders, Philadelphia, 70–75.
13. Page, D.L., Dupont, W.D., Rogers, L.W., Rados, M.S. (1985). Atypical hyperplastic lesions of the female breast: a long term follow-up study. *Cancer*, **55**, 2698–2708.
14. Page, D.L., Dupont, W.D., Rogers, L.W. (1988). Ductal involvement by cells of atypical lobular hyperplasia in the breast: a long term follow-up study of cancer risk. *Hum. Path.*, **19**, 201–207.
15. Page, D.L., Dupont, W.D., Rogers, L.W., Landenberger, M. (1982). Intraductal carcinoma of the breast: follow-up after biopsy only. *Cancer*, **49**, 751–758.
16. Rosen, P.P., Lieberman, P.H., Braun, D.W. Jr, *et al.* (1978). Lobular carcinoma *in situ* of the breast: detailed analysis of 99 patients with average follow-up of 24 years. *Amer. J. Surg. Path.*, **2**, 225–251.
17. Haagensen, C.D., Lane, N., Lattes, R. *et al.* (1978). Lobular neoplasia (so-called lobular carcinoma *in situ*) of the breast. *Cancer*, **42**, 737–769.
18. Silverstein, M.J., Rosser, R.J., Gierson, E.D. *et al.* (1987). Axillary lymph node dissection for intraductal breast carcinoma – Is it indicated? *Cancer*, **59**, 1819–1824.
19. Lagios, M.D., Westdahl, P.R., Margolin, F.R. *et al.* (1982). Duct carcinoma *in situ*. Relationship of extent of noninvasive disease to the frequency of occult invasion, multicentricity, lymph node metastases, and short-term treatment failures. *Cancer*, **50**, 1309-1314.
20. Schnitt, S.J., Silen, W., Sadowsky, N.L. *et al.* (1988). Ductal carcinoma *in situ* (intraductal carcinoma) of the breast. *New Engl. J. Med.*, **318**, 898–903.
21. Kelsey, J.L., Hildreth, N.G., Thompson, W.D. (1983). Epidemiologic aspects of breast cancer. *Radio. Clin. N. Amer.*, **21**, 3–12.
22. DuPont, W.D., Page, D.L. (1987). Breast cancer risk associated with proliferative disease, age at first birth, and a family history of breast cancer. *Amer. J. Epidem.*, **125**, 769–779.
23. MacMahon, B., Cole, P., Lin, T.M. *et al.* (1970). Age at first birth and breast cancer risk. *Bull. World, Hlth. Org.*, **43**, 209–221.
24. Odenheimer, D.J., Zunzunegui, M.V., King, M.C. *et al.* (1984). Risk factors for benign breast disease: a case-control study of discordant twins. *Amer. J. Epidem.*, **120**, 565–571.
25. Boyle, C.A., Berkowitz, G.S., LiVolsi, V.A. *et al.* (1984). Caffeine consumption and fibrocystic breast disease: a case-control epidemiologic study. *J. Nat. Cancer Inst.*, **72**, 1015–1019.
26. Li Volsi, V.A., Stadel, B.V., Kelsey, J.L. *et al.* (1978). Fibrocystic breast disease in oral-contraceptive users: a histopathological evaluation of epithelial atypia. *N. Engl. J. Med.*, **299**, 381–385.

27. Wolf, J.N. (1976). Risk for breast cancer development determined by mammographic parenchymal pattern. *Cancer*, **37**, 2486–2492.
28. Saftlas, A.F., Syklo, M. (1987). Mammographic parenchymal patterns and breast cancer risk. *Epidem. Rev.*, **9**, 146–174.
29. Boyd, N.F., O'Sullivan, B., Fishell, E. *et al.* (1984). Mammographic patterns and breast cancer risk: methodologic standard and contradictory results. *J. Nat. Cancer Inst.*, **72**, 1253–1259.
30. Gravelle, I.H., Bulstrode, R.D., Wang, D.Y. *et al.* (1986). A prospective study of mammographic parenchymal patterns and risk of breast cancer. *Brit. J. Radiol.*, **59**, 487–491.
31. Bright, R.A., Morrison, A.S., Brisson, J. *et al.* (1988). Relationship between mammographic and histologic features of breast tissue in women with benign biopsies. *Cancer*, **61**, 266–271.
32. Gold, R.H., Bassett, L.W., Kimme-Smith, C. (1986). Breast imaging: state-of-the-art. *Prog. Clin. Radiol.*, **21**, 298–304.

Chapter 6

Relationship to Diet and Body Size

STEPHANIE J. LONDON and WALTER C. WILLETT

Laboratory researchers have long known that diet influences the incidence of breast tumors in animals [1] but only recently has attention been focused on dietary factors in the causation and prevention of human breast cancer. The link between breast cancer and diet was suggested by findings of large international differences in breast cancer incidence rates. Thus, the age-adjusted incidence rates of breast cancer are five times higher in the United States and other Western industralized nations than in many other countries, while a low incidence is more typical of the generally less developed countries of Asia, Africa and Latin America. Although Japan, a country with low incidence, may appear to be an exception to this pattern, it had a largely agrarian population until relatively recently.

Studies of migrant populations have shown that genetic factors do not explain the large international variations in breast cancer incidence, because populations migrating from an area of low incidence tend to acquire rates characteristic of the new area (see Chapter 2). Moreover, changes in incidence rates over time in genetically stable populations show that often factors influence the incidence of breast cancer. Of such factors, diet may be responsible for 50% of all breast cancer in the United States [2] and the challenge is to identify which dietary factors are important and to quantify their effects.

Dietary Fat and Risk

Recent recommendations to reduce fat consumption [3] are based in part on the publication of striking correlations between national *per capita* fat consumption and both incidence and mortality rates of breast cancer [4]. Because the international differences in breast cancer rates are particularly great for postmenopausal women, diet is postulated to be most strongly associated with breast cancer among these women [5]. As a result, despite a relative paucity of analytic data in humans to support the hypothesis, a committee of the National Research Council has issued a provisional recommendation that the fat content of the US diet be reduced from an average of 40% to an average of 30% of calories, largely based on an anticipated reduction in breast cancer rates [6]. This has subsequently become the focus of a major health promotion campaign by the National Cancer Institute in the United States. The scientific basis for the recommendation is reviewed below.

Correlational Studies

Correlational studies involve comparisons of disease rates in different populations with their *per capita* consumption of specific dietary factors and such studies have several strengths. One is the strong contrasts produced. For example, in the US most individuals derive between 30 and 45% of their calories from fat, whereas the mean fat intake in different countries ranges from approximately 11 to 42% of calories [7]. Again, the average diets of different countries are likely to have been more stable for longer periods of time than the diets of individuals within a study. Finally, the cancer rates on which the studies are based are usually derived from large populations and therefore are more likely to be precise.

The main weakness of correlational studies is that established risk factors for breast cancer, other than fat intake, may differ between countries with high and low rates of the disease. For example, high incidence countries tend to be Westernized while low incidence countries tend to be non-industrialized, so that gross national product correlates as strongly with breast cancer mortality as does fat intake. Risk factors for breast cancer, such as low parity and late age at first birth, are more common in Westernized countries, and might be responsible for much of the apparent association between dietary fat and breast cancer risk. Another serious limitation of international correlational studies is the use of *per capita* dietary data that are only indirectly related to an individual intake because to some extent, they probably represent a relationship between food *wastage* and breast cancer risk.

In contrast to the strong correlation between *per capita* fat intake and breast cancer incidence, other correlational data are less striking. A positive correlation between *per capita* consumption of dairy fat and breast cancer rates has been noted for geographic areas within England, but fat intake from other sources was *inversely* related to breast cancer rates [8]. Within the US, regional consumption of milk (an important fat source) is positively associated with rates of breast cancer, although consumption of eggs (a major cholesterol determinant) is *inversely* related to breast cancer rates [9].

It has been shown that the offspring of immigrants from Japan to the United States, (but not the immigrants themselves) have breast cancer rates that are similar to those of the general American population [10], while Polish women who migrate to the United States quickly attain rates of breast cancer that are similar to the higher rates among US-born women [11]. It may be that the delayed effect among Japanese Americans is due to a slower acculturation process (see Chapter 2).

Special Populations

It was originally reported that, compared to the general US population, breast cancer mortality rates were lower among Seventh-Day Adventists, who consume relatively small amounts of meat and other animal products [12]. However, when compared to a US white population of *similar socio-economic level* breast cancer mortality rates among a large group of Seventh-Day Adventists were found to be only slightly and non-significantly lower than expected [13]. Although total fat intake of Seventh-Day Adventists is not particularly low, vegetable fat is largely substituted for animal fat; thus, these data do not support the hypothesis that animal fat or meat intake are specifically related to breast cancer. Moreover, among Seventh-Day Adventists, women following a vegetarian diet for a longer period tended to have a non-significantly higher breast cancer mortality than women following such a diet for a shorter period [14].

Rates of breast cancer among orders of nuns who were either vegetarians or ate only small amounts of meat have been compared with rates among single British women but no significant differences were found [15]. The very strong correlation between dietary fat intake and breast cancer rates among five ethnic groups living in Hawaii [16] has been interpreted by some as evidence of a causal relationship. However, the implausibly strong relationship between dietary fats and breast cancer risk seen in this data (much stronger than suggested by the international correlations) suggests that the association observed in this study is confounded by some other factors.

Changes Over Time

Dramatic changes in breast cancer incidence in Iceland during this century provide further strong evidence of non-genetic factors [17]. The diet of the Icelandic population has changed substantially over that period of time, becoming high in fat content like other Western countries. These data are consistent with the hypothesis that high fat intake causes breast cancer, but do not exclude other possible explanations. In Japan, too, fat intake has increased dramatically since World War II, from about 10% of calories to about 25% of calories by 1975. However, age-adjusted breast cancer mortality and incidence rates increased much less markedly [18, 19]. While these data do not suggest a major role of dietary fat intake in breast cancer etiology, the full impact of the dramatic dietary changes in Japan might not be seen for several more decades if diet acts primarily during childhood.

Consumption of different types of fats has been related to the apparent increase in incidence of breast and other cancers in the United States [20]. It is reported that the strongest association is that with the consumption of *trans*-fatty acids, which are fatty acids created in processes that convert liquid vegetable oils to margarine and solid vegetable shortening. However, it is not clear whether the US incidence of breast cancer has actually been increasing beyond what would be expected on the basis of a trend toward later and fewer pregnancies. Sudden changes in national diets due to war and social upheavals may potentially be useful to examine the latent period between change in diet and change in breast cancer rates. Although intake of meat and fat declined during World War II in England, there was no important decline in breast cancer mortality [21].

Case-control Studies

In such studies, information regarding previous diet is obtained from patients with breast cancer and compared to that of subjects without the disease. In a case-control study of this relationship, Miller *et al.* [22] compared the diets of 400 Canadian women with breast cancer with those of 400 neighborhood controls and concluded that their data showed an association between dietary fat and breast cancer. However, a careful review of the paper suggests that this is not the case. In this study, three methods were used to assess dietary intake: (1) a recall of foods consumed within the past 24 hours; (2) a 4-day diet record; and (3) a dietary history questionnaire referring to a period before diagnosis. In their companion paper, the authors stated appropriately that the dietary history is inherently more reliable than either of the first two methods [23]. Furthermore, they correctly note that in a case-control study there is reason to be concerned that the diagnosis or treatment of cancer could alter diet or its recall: another reason why the dietary history should be superior. However, the only significant findings in the paper are based on the 24-hour recall. Moreover, the results are not adjusted for caloric intake. When fat intake is calculated as a percentage of total calories, it is seen that the cases reported 39.1% of calories from fat compared to 39.0% for controls. For saturated fat the values are 15% for cases and 15.1% for controls. Clearly, these are not significant differences. Thus, this carefully executed study actually provides no support for the hypothesis that the fat composition of the diet affects the risk of breast cancer.

The largest case-control study to date of dietary fat intake and breast cancer incidence was reported by Graham *et al.* [24]. Fat intake estimated with a simple food frequency questionnaire among 2024 women with breast cancer was essentially identical to that reported by 1463 control women attending a hospital for a variety of benign conditions.

All US and Canada studies share the constraint that few women consume a diet with less than 30% of calories derived from fat. For this reason the Japanese case-control study of Hirohata *et al.* [25] conduced among 212 women with breast cancer and an equal number each of hospitalized and neighborhood controls is of special interest. In this study, the mean daily total fat intake reported by cases was 51 grams, by hospital controls was 52, and by neighborhood controls was 52, and lack of any substantial difference was seen for both animal fat and vegetable fat. A similar lack of association between fat intake and breast cancer risk was observed in a small case-control study conducted in Greece [26].

A number of other case-control studies of breast cancer have investigated the use of specific high-fat foods, but were not extensive enough to provided an estimate of total fat intake. One of these studies [27], has frequently been cited as supporting the hypothesis linking fat and breast cancer. Data on cases and controls were not obtained in a comparable manner: a serious problem in case-control studies which may lead to a biased result. Striking associations were found for the use of beef, port, and sweet deserts. However, these findings are *not* consistent with the results of studies in Seventh-Day Adventists, or vegetarian nuns, or of the case-control studies of Graham and Miller, or of the prospective studies discussed below.

Prospective Studies

Of the prospective studies published, Phillips and Snowdon [28] examined the relationship between meat consumption and mortality due to breast cancer during a 21-year follow-up of California Seventh-Day Adventists. During this period 186 women died of this disease and no significant trend in breast cancer mortality was found for increasing meat consumption. These data are of particular value because of the large portion of the population that consumed no meat at all. In the first large prospective study reported, calculation of total fat intake was based on a dietary questionnaire completed by 89 523 registered nurses aged 34 to 59 years in 1980 [29]. During four years of follow-up, 601 cases of breast cancer were diagnosed among the participants. After adjustments for known determinants of breast cancer, no elevation in the risk of breast cancer was found for increased total fat, saturated fat, lineoleic acid, cholesterol or meat intake. Indeed, non-significant *decrease* in risk was seen for women with the highest consumption of total and saturated fat.

This study was unique because it included a validation study that provided a measurement of the distribution of fat intake in the study population independent of the study questionnaire. Based on 28 days of diet records completed by 173 participants, the mean values for lowest and highest categories of fat intake range from 32 to 44% of total calories. Ideally, it would be of considerable interest to examine the effect of fat intake below 30% of calories; however, these data suggest that this will be difficult in a contemporary general US population since relatively few people eat so little fat. Nevertheless, the degree of variation in fat intake within the study population is of interest since it corresponds closely to the current advice to decrease fat intake by one fourth from an average of 40% calories to 30% of calories, and is therefore sufficient to evaluate the effect of these recommendations. For saturated fat intake which is most highly suspected because of the international correlations, the variation in intake was greater.

This prospective study of US nurses provides evidence against the hypothesis that dietary fat intake, within the range consumed by the general US population, causes breast cancer. However, the possibility that a more severe fat restriction to well below 30% of total calories might decrease the risk to breast cancer could not be addressed. In addition, a dietary questionnaire is a good, but not perfect, measure of dietary fat intake.

Another recently reported prospective study, used a 24-hour recall provided by women collected as a part of a US nutritional survey to calculate fat intake [30]. Within the study population over 10 years of average follow-up 99 women developed breast cancer. The incidence rates were actually 50% lower among women with the highest total fat intake compared to those with the lowest fat intake, although this inverse relationship was no longer statistically significant after adjusting for total caloric intake.

In summary, the case-control and cohort studies that have been sufficiently comprehensive to allow a computation of total fat intake have been remarkably consistent in failing to provide evidence of a positive association between the dietary lipid content and risk of breast cancer. Sporadic associations have been observed between meat and dairy products in some case-control studies with a limited dietary assessment. However, these associations have not been consistently observed in these limited studies or the more comprehensive case-control studies, and are inconsistent with the rates of breast cancer in Seventh-Day Adventists [13] and vegetarian nuns [15]. Moreover, if true, these positive associations with meat intake should have been readily observable in the prospective studies of Phillips and Snowdon [28], Willett *et al.* [29], and Jones [30]. It is thus most likely that these sporadic findings represent the play of chance combined with a tendency for positive associations to be reported.

Construction of a plausible mechanism whereby fat may affect the risk of breast cancer is seriously hindered by our basic ignorance of the pathophysiology of this disease. Support for the hypothesis that high levels of dietary fat increase the rate of breast cancer is derived from studies that have related dietary factors to estrogen fractions and levels of other hormones, which are, in turn, thought to be related to breast cancer risk [31]. However, the results have not been consistent and the relationship between levels of specific hormones and the risk of breast cancer has not been firmly established (see Chapter 4).

Again, the hypothesis that high-fat diets cause breast cancer in humans has been based on animal studies but the interpretation of these laboratory findings is controversial. This issue is discussed at length by Birt [32] and in the proceedings of a recent symposium [33] Albanes [34] performed a meta-analysis of mammary cancer experiments in mice conducted over the past 50 years and found an extremely strong overall positive association between breast cancer and high total energy intake while fat composition was weakly *inversely* related to incidence of mammary tumors after adjustment for total energy intake. Yet, Birt has concluded that evidence does exist for an effect of fat independent of energy intake [32]. It is clear that restriction of energy intake dramatically lowers the incidence of mammary tumors in animals, but a central question is whether fat intake has an effect on mammary cancer independent of its substantial contribution to total energy intake.

The failure of most case-control and cohort studies to confirm the hypothesis that a diet high in total or saturated fat composition increases the incidence of human breast cancer leaves the large differences in breast cancer rates among countries unexplained. Many alternative hypotheses exist, including the differences in intake of selenium and other minerals [35], marine oils [36], alcohol [37, 38] and specific vegetables [39, 40]. Evidence for these hypothesis will be reviewed later in this chapter.

Body Size and Risk

Indices of body size, such as height and relative weight have been extensively studied in relation to the risk of breast cancer. The positive relationship between energy intake and mammary cancer seen in animals has led to the hypothesis that energy restriction sufficient to restrict adult height may decrease the risk of breast cancer, and De Waard found a strong correlation (similar in magnitude for that seen for dietary fat consumption) between average national heights and breast cancer incidence [4]. However, height is not a good measure in all populations of energy intake during development. Where food is widely available, such as in the US and other Western industralized countries, it is unlikely than many individuals experience sufficient energy restriction to limit growth. In these populations, height is primarily under genetic control. In contrast, in other societies, height does not reflect nutritional factors and an example is Japan where a major increase in height has occurred in this century coincident with industrialization [18].

Studies of height and the risk of breast cancer among individuals (case-control and prospective studies) support this dichotomy between the use of height as a measure of energy intake in societies in which caloric deprivation has or has not been widespread. In general, increased height is not associated with increased risk of breast cancer in Western industralized countries such as the US [42] and Sweden [43]. In contrast, taller women have been found to be at increased risk in studies in countries where major portions of the population are likely to have experienced caloric restriction in this century such as Japan [44] and Greece [45].

Relative body weight, has been even more widely studied in relation to the risk of breast cancer. Weight is rarely used alone among adults since it relates to both height and body composition. Obesity, in contrast to height, does provide a sensitive indicator of energy intake in excess of energy expenditure during adulthood. Early epidemiologic data suggested that high relative weight increased the risk of breast cancer but more recent data indicate that the association is far more complex than originally appreciated. In interpreting the data, prospective data are preferable to case-control data but there have been few prospective studies. In addition, studies in which a positive association was found were often those in which menopausal status was not considered, yet recent data suggest that relative body weight is likely to relate differently to premenopausal and postmenopausal breast cancer. In a number of studies in which menopausal status was taken into account, including one large prospective study [42], *leaner* women have been found to be at increased risk of breast cancer during the premenopausal years [46, 47]. A similar association has also been seen for relative weight at age 18 [42]; a finding which further increases the complexity of this relationship. After the menopause, the data generally demonstrate a modest increase in risk with higher relative weight only among the older postmenopausal women [48, 46, 47].

In a large prospective study, in which menopausal status was not considered, a modest overall increase in risk was seen for obese women, but the endpoint was breast cancer mortality, not incidence as in the other studies cited [49]. Obese women may have a higher breast cancer mortality as a result of delayed detection of breast cancer in a large breast, while lean women are more likely to show smaller tumors at the time of diagnosis. Although this could lead to a bias in prospective studies of incidence, it is unlikely that the effect of leanness seen among premenopausal women, in the prospective study of Willett *et al.* results solely from detection bias [42].

In summary, the data suggest that energy restriction sufficient to reduce height may reduce the risk of breast cancer. However, even if this association does explain some of the international differences in breast cancer rates, it does not have direct implications for breast cancer prevention. Caloric restriction in children sufficient to stunt growth is neither practical nor desirable. Furthermore, the data on relative weight suggest that such an intervention might actually increase the risk of breast cancer in premenopausal women. Although many mechanisms have been postulated by which obesity might increase the risk of breast cancer, the available data suggest that it is at most a modest risk factor and has its effect only on older postmenopausal women. Thus, even major success in controlling obesity would achieve only very minor reductions in the incidence of breast cancer.

Micronutrients and Risk

Vitamin A

The term vitamin A refers to the combination of preformed vitamin A (retinol and related compounds) and carotenoids with provitamin A activity. Among the carotenoids, beta-carotene has the highest provitamin A activity and has been the most widely studied with respect to cancer incidence. Experimental evidence in animals suggests a role for vitamin A in prevention of cancer and both retinol and beta-carotene have antioxidant activity. In general, the animal data is stronger for retinol but the study of beta-carotene may be more difficult in rodents because its absorption into the blood is low in comparison to humans [50]. In the human there are relatively few studies on the relationship between dietary vitamin A intake and the risk of breast cancer. Data from two case-control studies demonstrate a higher risk of breast cancer in women with lower consumption of foods containing vitamin A [24, 26].

To assess the relationship between vitamin A and breast cancer incidence, some investigators have measured serum levels of vitamin A. Because cancer may lower blood levels of vitamin A (as well as other nutrients) the finding of diminished levels of either retinol or carotenoids in breast cancer patients cannot be interpreted as evidence that low levels caused the disease. Data from two small prospective studies does not show a relationship between the risk of developing breast cancer and prediagnostic levels of retinol or beta-carotene [51, 52]. However, the possibility that vitamin A intake has an effect on breast cancer incidence is by no means ruled out by these studies: serum retinol is not a sensitive marker of vitamin A intake in generally well-nourished populations. Furthermore, it is possible that a component of green and yellow vegetables (major sources of carotenoids), other than beta-carotene, is protective for breast cancer. In support of this hypotheses, one study found stronger protective associations for individual vegetables, especially carrots, than for vitamin A intake as a whole [26, 53].

Vitamin E

A possible role of vitamin E in cancer prevention has been suggested based on its role as an antioxidant. However, there is limited data in animals or humans to support a protective role for either its intake or blood levels of vitamin E [51]. In the two studies in which serum vitamin E was measured before diagnosis, low levels were associated with increased risk of breast cancer in one [52], but not in the other [51]. Unlike the case of retinol, vitamin E levels do closely reflect intake.

Vitamin C

There are few data on the relationship between vitamin C intake and the risk of breast cancer in humans and no association was seen in two case-control studies [24, 26]. Although vitamin C blocks formation of carcinogenic nitrosamines in people and animals, more general evidence of an anticarcinogenic effect is lacking [50].

Selenium

Selenium is an essential trace element that plays a key role in the activity of glutathione peroxidase, an enzyme that protects cells against damage from oxidizing chemicals. Correlation studies have provided evidence to suggest a role for selenium in cancer prevention: geographic areas with low selenium levels in the soil or in pooled blood bank samples generally have higher cancer rates than do areas with higher selenium levels [35]. However, this type of data must be interpreted with caution since high selenium areas in the US are sparsely populated areas which differ in many respects from low selenium areas, which include the major urban centers.

Intake of selenium cannot be assessed accurately by questionnaire because the selenium content of a given food varies widely. In contrast, intake can be assessed using blood or toenail measurements. As is true of measurements of other nutrients, cancer may decrease levels of selenium in the blood, therefore studies in which samples were collected before the diagnosis of cancer are most valuable. No difference between selenium measurements in breast cancer cases compared with controls was found in two prospective studies [54, 55], although the risk of all types of cancer combined decreased with increasing levels of selenium [55]. Since neither study had large numbers of women with breast cancer, a true association could have been missed.

Alcohol and Coffee Intake

Epidemiologic data linking alcohol intake to the risk of breast cancer demonstrate remarkable consistency. A positive association has been found in most studies including three prospective studies [37, 38, 56] and a large case-control study [57]. The association is not explained by established breast cancer risk factors nor by other dietary factors. Among women in a large prospective study, those who drank two to three drinks per week experienced a 40% increase in risk; those who drank one or more drinks per day experienced a 50% increase in risk [37]. The finding of a dose response relationship increases the likelihood that the association between moderate alcohol intake and breast cancer is indeed causal.

In one study in which data on alcohol intake at difference ages was collected, the adverse consequences of alcohol intake related to drinking practices before age 30;

current drinking did not increase the risk of breast cancer [57]. Most studies have not included information on drinking throughout life. If this finding were confirmed in other studies, it would imply that young women might decrease their risk of breast cancer by curtailing even moderate alcohol intake but that older women would not. Given the possible beneficial effects of moderate alcohol intake on cardiovascular disease (a problem more common in older women) this information carries great public health importance. Thus, until more data are available, the finding that moderate alcohol intake increases the risk of breast cancer does not readily translate into advice to middle-aged women on whether to curtail moderate alcohol intake.

It is difficult to explain the effect of alcohol on breast cancer incidence although alcohol readily permeates breast tissue and is clearly implicated as a cause of cancer in the gastrointestinal tract. Alcohol has been found to affect release of prolactin. In addition, it can increase lipid peroxidation in some circumstances and therefore may lead to DNA damage by free radicals. These facts may provide possible explanations for the epidemiologic evidence [37].

Reports that some women with breast pain may experience resolution of symptoms after abstention from coffee has led to the hypothesis that coffee may be a cause of benign breast disease [58]. Again, since some types of benign breast disease lead to increased risk of breast cancer, it has been hypothesized that coffee may increase the risk of breast cancer. However, the association between coffee and benign breast disease is not well established and although the risk of breast cancer in relation to coffee drinking has been investigated in several studies, there is little evidence to support an association. No association was found in a prospective study of Seventh-Day Adventists [59] nor in a large case-control study [58].

Diet and Prognosis

Traditionally, Japanese women have shown higher breast cancer survival rates [60] as well as lower incidence rates compared to US women [61] but as Japan has become more Westernized, breast cancer mortality has increased more rapidly than have incidence rates [61]. While Japanese patients tend to be diagnosed at an earlier stage of disease, they have improved survival rates compared to US women even after controlling for stage of disease at diagnosis [60] which suggests that environmental factors, notably diet, may influence breast cancer prognosis. In spite of this, Japanese-born migrants are found to have comparable survival rats to second-generation Japanese in Hawaii [62].

Obesity has been widely studied in relation to breast cancer survival but the data are inconclusive. Obesity was found to be associated with increased recurrence in one study, but no trend with increasing levels of obesity was seen [63]. Boyd [64] found a significant association only in women with stage 1 breast cancer and the overall association was reduced after adjustment for stage at diagnosis. Sohrabi [65] found no association between obesity and time to recurrence. In interpreting these studies, it is important to note that more obese women are likely to present with larger tumors and with nodal metastases [42]. Since tumor size and nodal metastases are strong predictors of recurrence, an apparent association between obesity and breast cancer prognosis might be due to the association between obesity and stage at diagnosis.

Dietary fat has been little studied in relation to breast cancer prognosis. In one study, fat intake was associated with recurrence only in women with distant metastases [66]. Zollinger [67] found no difference in survival between Seventh-Day Adventist women (more than half of whom do not eat meat) and other white Californians after adjusting for an earlier stage at diagnosis among the Adventists. While available data do not support a powerful effect of dietary fat on prognosis, much larger studies would be needed to detect a modest effect. Recently, a large trial in the US was discontinued due to insufficient numbers of patients willing to adhere to a highly fat-restricted diet, and there is no evidence at present that women with breast cancer should reduce their intake of dietary fats.

Conclusion

At present, the large variation in the incidence of breast cancer across the world remains unexplained. The hypothesis that fat intake increases the risk of breast cancer is based largely on international correlation studies and is generally not supported by the rest of the available data despite a large number of case-control and three prospective studies. This suggests that the current recommendations to American women to decrease their fat intake by 25% is not likely to result in a decrease in breast cancer incidence despite other possible healthy benefits. However, it cannot be excluded that more severe fat restriction may have some impact on breast cancer risk.

Specific fatty acids, notably the marine oils, may be related to the risk of breast cancer and have been little investigated in humans. The hypothesis that caloric restriction sufficient to decrease height may decrease the risk of breast cancer is supported by several lines of investigation, but does not have practical implications for prevention.

Among the micronutrients, the possibility that vitamin A exerts a protective effect merits further investigation, and similarly, the role of selenium has not been sufficiently explored. If these factors were found to be beneficial, they could be readily supplemented in the diet.

Of the dietary factors studied to date, moderate alcohol intake most consistently emerges as a risk factor for breast cancer. Since this is the only readily modifiable risk factor that has been identified, data are needed to determine whether cessation of drinking will decrease a woman's risk of breast cancer or lessen the likelihood of a recurrence.

References

1. Tannenbaum, A. (1942). The genesis and growth of tumors, III. Effects of a high fat diet. *Cancer Res.*, **2**, 468–475.
2. Doll, R., Peto, R. (1981). The causes of cancer; quantitative estimates of avoidable risks of cancer in the United States. *J. Nat. Cancer Inst.*, **66**, 1191-1308.
3. Willett, W.C. (1988). *Methods in Nutritional Epidemiology*, Oxford University Press, New York.
4. Armstrong, B., Doll, R. (1975). Environmental factors and cancer incidence and mortality in different countries, with special reference to dietary practices. *Int. J. Cancer*, **15**, 617–631.
5. de Waard, F., Baanders-van Halewijn, E. A., Huizinga, J. (1964). The bimodal age distribution of patients with mammary carcinoma: evidence for the existence of two types of human breast cancer. *Cancer*, **17**, 141–151.
6. National Research Council, Committee on Diet, Nutrition and Cancer (1982). *Diet, Nutrition, and Cancer*, National Academy Press, Washington, D.C.
7. Hebert, J.R., Wynder, E.L. (1987). Dietary fat and the risk of breast cancer (letter). *N. Engl. J. Med.*, **317**, 165.
8. Stocks, P. (1970). Breast cancer anomalies. *Brit. J. Cancer*, **24**, 633–643.
9. Gaskill, S.P., McGuire, W.L., Osborne, C.K., Stern, M.P. (1979). Breat cancer mortality and diet in the United States. *Cancer Res.*, **39**, 3628–3637.
10. Buell, P. (1973). Changing incidence of breast cancer in Japanese-American women. *J. Nat. Cancer Inst.*, **51**, 1479–1483.
11. Staszewski, J., Haenszel, W. (1965). Cancer mortality among the Polish-born in the United States. *J. Nat. Cancer Inst.*, **35**, 291–297.
12. Phillips, R.L. (1975). Role of life-style and dietary habits in risk of cancer among Seventh-Day Adventists. *Cancer Res.*, **35**, 3513–3522.
13. Phillips R.L., Garfinkel, L., Beeson, J.W., Lotz, T., Brin, B. (1980). Mortality among California Seventh-Day Adventists for selected cancer sites. *J. Nat. Cancer Inst.*, **65**, 1097–1107.
14. Mills, P.K., Annegers, J.F., Phillips, R.L. (1988). Animal product consumption and subsequent fatal breast cance risk among Seventh-Day Adventist women. *Amer. J. Epidem.*, **127**, 440–453.
15. Kinlen, L.J. (1982). Meat and fat consumption and cancer mortality: a study of strict regligious orders in Britain. *Lancet*, **i**, 946–949.
16. Kolonel, L.N., Hankin, J.H., Nomura, A.M., Chu, S.Y. (1981). Dietary fat intake and cancer incidence among five ethnic groups in Hawaii. *Cancer Res.*, **41**, 327–328.
17. Bjarnason, O., Day, N., Snaedal, G., Tulinius, H. (1974). The effect of year of birth on the breast cancer age-incidence curve in Iceland. *Int. J. Cancer*, **13**, 689–696.
18. Hirayama, T. (1978). Epidemiology of breast cancer with special reference to the role of diet. *Prev. Med.*, **7**, 173–195.
19. Hanai, A., Fujimoto, I. (1982). Cancer incidence in Japan in 1975 and changes in epidemiologic features for cancer in Osaka. *Nat. Cancer Inst., Monograph 62*, 3–7.
20. Enig, M.G., Munn, R.J., Kenney, M. (1978). Dietary fat and cancer trends – a critique. *Fed. Proc.*, **37**, 2215–2220.
21. Key, T.J.A., Darby, S.C., Pike, M.C. (1987). Trends in breast cancer mortality and diet in England and Wales from 1911 to 1980. *Nutr. Cancer*, **10**, 1–10.
22. Miller, A.B., Kelly, A., Choi, N.W. *et al.* (1978). A study of diet and breast cancer. *Amer. J. Epidem.*, **107**, 499–509.

23. Morgan, R.W., Jain, M., Miller, A.B., Choi, N.W., Mathews, V., Munan, L., Burch, J.D., Feather, J., Howe, G., Kelly, A. (1978). A comparison of dietary methods in epidemiologic studies. *Amer. J. Epidem.*, **107**, 488–498.
24. Graham, S.J., Marshall, xx, Mettlin, C., Rzepka, T., Neomoto, T., Byers, T. (1982). Diet in the epidemiology of breast cancer. *Amer. J. Epidem.*, **116**, 68–75.
25. Hirohata, T., Shigematsu, T., Nomura, A.M.Y., Nomura, Y., Horie, A., Hirohata, I. (1985). Occurrence of breast cancer in relation to diet and reproductive history: a case-control study in Fukuoka, Japan. *Nat. Cancer Inst., Monograph 69*, 187–190.
26. Katsouyanni, K., Willett, W., Boyle, P., Trichopoulos, D., Vasilaros, S., Papadiamantis, J., MacMahon, B. (1987). Risk of breast cancer among Greek women in relation to nutrient intake. *Cancer*, **61**, 181–185.
27. Lubin, J.H., Burns, P.E., Blot, W.J., Ziegler, R.G., Lees, A.W., Fraumeni, J.R. Jr (1981). Dietary factors and breast cancer risk. *Int. J. Cancer*, **28**, 685–689.
28. Phillips, R.L., Snowdon, D.A. (1983). Association of meat and coffee use with cancers of the large bowel, breast, and prostate among Seventh-Day Adventists: preliminary results. *Cancer Res.*, **43**, 5: Suppl., 2403–2408.
29. Willett, W.C., Stampfer, M.J., Colditz, G.A., Rosner, B.A., Nennekens, C.H., Speizer, F.E. (1987). Dietary fat and risk of breast cancer. *N. Engl. J. Med.*, **316**, 22–28.
30. Jones, D.Y., Schatzkin, A., Green, S.B. *et al.* (1987). Dietary fat and breast cancer in the National Health and Nutrition Examination survey and epidemiologic follow-up study. *J. Nat. Cancer Inst.*, **79**, 465–471.
31. Willett, W.C., MacMahon, B. (1984). Diet and cancer – an overview. *N. Engl. J. Med.*, **310**, 633–638 and 607–701.
32. Birt, D.F. Dietary fat and experimental carcinogenesis: a summary of recent *in vivo* studies. In *Advances in Experimental Medicine and Biology: Essential Nutrients in Carcinogenesis*, Vol. 206, 69–84.
33. Pariza, M.W., Simopoulos, A.P. (eds.), (1987, Supplement). Calories and energy expenditure in carcinogenesis. *Amer. J. Clin. Nutr.*, **45**, 149–272.
34. Albanes, D. (1987). Total calories, body weight, and tumor incidence in mice. *Cancer Res.*, **47**, 1987–1992.
35. Shamberger, R.J., Tytko, S.A., Willis, C.E. (1976). Antioxidants and cancer. VI. Selenium and age-adjusted human cancer mortality. *Arch. Environ. Health*, **31**, 231–235.
36. Karmali, R.A. XX. Fatty acids: inhibition. *Am. J. Clin. Nutr.*, **45**, (Supplement), 225–229.
37. Willett, W.C., Stampfer, M.J., Colditz, G.A., Rosner, B.A., Hennekens, C.H., Speizer, F.E. (1987). Moderate alcohol consumption and the risk of breast cancer. *N. Engl. J. Med.*, **316**, 1174–1179.
38. Schatzkin, A., Jones, Y., Hoover, R.N. *et al.* (1987). Alcohol consumption and breast cancer in the epidemiologic follow-up study of the first National Health and Nutrition Examination Survey. *N. Engl. J. Med.*, **316**, 1169–1173.
39. Kamiyama, S., Michioka, O. (1983). Mutagenic components of diets in high and low-risk areas for stomach cancer. In: Stich, H.F. (ed.), *Carcinogens and Mutagens in the Environment*, CRC Press, Boca Raton, Fla, 29–42.
40. Knox, E.G. (1977). Foods and diseases. *Brit. J. Prev. Soc. Med.*, **31**, 71–80.
41. Breast-cancer incidence and nutritional status with particular reference to body weight and height. *Cancer Res.*, **35**, 3351–3356.
42. Willet, W.C., Browne, M.L., Bain, C. *et al.* (1985). Relative weight and risk of breast cancer among premenopausal women. Amer. J. Epidem., **122**, 731–740.
43. Adami, H.O., Rimsten, A., Stenkvist, B. *et al.* (1977). Influence of height, weight, and obesity on risk of breast cancer in an unselected Swedish population. *Brit. J. Cancer*, **36**, 787–792.

44. de Waard, F., Cornelis, J.P., Aoki, K., Yoshida, M. (1977). Breast cancer incidence according to weight and height in two cities in the Netherlands and in Aichi Prefecture, Japan. *Cancer*, **40**, 1269–1275.

45. Valaoras, V.G., MacMahon, B., Trichopoulos, D. *et al.* (1969). Lactation and reproductive histories of breast cancer patients in greater Athens, 1965–67. *Int. J. Cancer*, **4**, 350–363.

46. Hilsop, T.G., Coldman, A.J., Elwood, J.M., Brauer, G., Kan, L. (1986). Childhood and recent eating patterns and risk of breast cancer. *Cancer Detection and Prevention*, **9**, 47–58.

47. Choi, N.W., Howe, G.R., Miller, A.B., Matthews, V., Morgan, R.W., Munan, L., Bunch, J.D., Feather, J., Jain, M., Kelly, A. (1978). An epidemiologic study of breast cancer. *Amer. J. Epidem.*, **107**, 510–521.

48. Lubin, F., Ruder, A.M., Wax, Y. Modan, B. (1985). Overweight and changes in weight throughout adult life in breast cancer etiology. *Amer. J. Epidem.*, **122**, 579–588.

49. Lew, E.A., Garfinkel, L. (1979). Variations in mortality by weight among 750,000 men and women. *J. Chron. Dis.*, **32**, 563–576.

50. Rogers, A.E., Longnecker, M.P. (in press). Dietary and nutritional influences in cancer: a review of the epidemiologic and experimental data. *Lab. Rev.*

51. Willett, W.C., Polk, F., Underwood, B.A. *et al.* (1984). Relation of serum vitamins A and E and carotenoids to the risk of cancer. *N. Engl. J. Med.*, **310**, 430-434.

52. Wald, N.J., Boreham, J., Hayward, J.L., Bulbrook, R.D. (1984). Plasma retinol, B-carotene and vitamin E levels in realtion to the future risk of breast cancer. *Brit. J. Cancer*, **49**, 321–324.

53. Katsouyanni, K., Trichopoulos, D., Boyle, P., Xironchaki, E., Trichopoulou, A., Lisseos, B., Basilaros, S., MacMahon, B. (1986). Diet and breast cancer: a case-control study in Greece. *Int. J. Cancer*, **38**, 815–820.

54. Van Noord, P.A.H., Collette, H.J.A., Maas, M.J., De Waard, F. (1987). Selenium levels in nails of premenopausal breast cancer patients assessed prediagnostically in a cohort-nested case-referent study among women screened in the DOM project. *Int. J. Epidem.*, **16**, (Suppl.), 318–322.

55. Willett, W.C., Polk, B.F., Morris, S.J., Stampfer, M.S. *et al.* (1983). Prediagnostic screen selenium and risk of cancer. *Lancet*, **ii**, 130–134.

56. Hiatt, R.A., Bawol, R.D. (1984). Alcholic Beverage consumption and breast cancer incidence. *Amer. J. Epidem.*, **120**, 676–683.

57. Harvey, E.B., Schairer, C., Brinton, L.A., Hoover, R.N., Fraumeni, J.F. (1987). Alcohol consumption and breast cancer. *J. Nat. Cancer Inst.*, **78**, 657–661.

58. Rosenberg, L., Miller, D.R., Helmrich, S.P., Kaufman, D.W., Schottenfeld, D., Stolley, P., Shapiro, S. (1985). Breast cancer and the consumption of coffee. *Amer. J. Epidem.*, **122**, 391–399.

59. Snowdon, D.A., Phillips, R.L. (1984). Coffee consumption and risk of fatal cancers. *Amer. J. Publ. Hlth.*, **74**, 820–823.

60. Morrison, A.S., Black, M.M., Lowe, C.R., MacMahon, B., Yuasa, S. (1973). Some international differences in histology and survival in breast cancer. *Int. J. Cancer*, **11**, 261–267.

61. Fujimoto, I., Hanai, A., Oshima, A. (1978). Description epidemiology of cancer in Japan: current cancer incidence and survival data. *Nat. Cancer Inst., Monograph 53*, 5–15.

62. LeMarchand, L., Kolonel, L.N., Nomura, A.M.Y. (1985). Breast cancer survival among Hawaii Japanese and Caucasian women. *Amer. J. Epidem.*, **122**, 571–578.

63. Donegan, W.L., Hartz, A.J., Rimm, A.A. (1978). The association of body weight with recurrent cancer of the breast. *Cancer*, **1**, 1590–1594.

64. Boyd, N.F., Campbell, J.E., Germanson, T., Thompson, D.B., Southerland, D.J., Meakin, J.W. (1981). Body weight and prognosis in breast cancer. *J. Nat. Cancer Inst.*, **67**, 785–789.

65. Sohrabi, A., Sandoz, XX, Spratt, J.S., Polk, H.C. (1980). Recurrence of breast cancer: obesity, tumor size and axillary lymph node metastases. *J. Amer. Med. Ass.*, **244**, 264–265.

66. Gregorio, D.I., Emrich, L.J., Graham, S., Marshall, J.R., Nemoto, T. (1985). Dietary fat consumption and survival among women with breast cancer. *J. Nat. Cancer Inst.*, **75**, 37–41.
67. Zollinger, T.W., Phillips, R.L., Kuzma, J.W. (1984). Breast cancer survival rates among Seventh-Day Adventists and non-Seventh-Day Adventists. *Amer. J. Epidem.*, **119**, 503–509.

Part Two

An Individualised Approach to Control

Chapter 7

Calculating a Woman's Degree of Risk

A.B. MILLER and M.T. SCHECHTER

Introduction

This chapter considers three aspects of breast cancer risk in women. The first relates to an individual woman's degree of risk for developing breast cancer during her lifetime. This knowledge will guide her and her medical advisors on how much effort she should apply to measures that might reduce her risk of breast cancer. The second relates to the importance in the population of the various risk factors for breast cancer and the proportion of deaths from breast cancer that might be averted by screening, if specific programmes were directed to each risk factor.

It is important to distinguish the two approaches. In the first, we are interested in the *relative* risk, that is the extent that an individual with that risk factor is at greater risk than someone without it. For example, we know that the degree of risk for an individual woman varies according to various aspects of her family history and her age. For some women, the *relative* risk from her family history may be as high as nine or more while for others there is no increase in risk. In the second approach, we are interested in the amount of breast cancer in the population, the risk *attributable* to a family history of breast cancer is of the order of 10%, and therefore may be of less concern for public health planners than, for example, the amount of breast cancer *attributable* to dietary fat intake, that could amount to 25% or more.

The third and fourth areas draw on both the preceding (but at present, particularly the first) in attempting to calculate the extent to which knowledge on risk factors can be combined, in relation to the individual woman, and in deciding whether or not women should participate in screening programmes. The fifth relates to the extent to which factors in a woman's history or background affect the outcome of treatment in women who have breast cancer.

The Importance of Various Risk Factors: the Individual Approach

The most important risk factor for breast cancer is age. For women born in Western Europe or North America the risk of breast cancer increases progressively with increasing age. Thus, a women in her eighties has about a 50% greater risk of developing breast cancer than a woman in her seventies (a relative risk – RR – of 1.5), and a woman in her seventies has about a 20% greater risk of developing breast cancer than a woman in her sixties (an RR of 1.2). Women in North America now have a *lifetime* risk of developing breast cancer of 9% (1 in 11), providing they do not die of another cause before age 75. The lifetime risk in Western Europe is a little lower.

The other major risk factor is being born in North America or Western Europe. Such women have an RR of breast cancer of 5 compared to women born, for example, in Japan. However, if women migrate from Japan to North America, they acquire a similar risk to North Americans over two or three generations. Acculturation to the North American life-style appears to have increased their risk (see Chapter 2).

Table 1 Relative risks for various factors

Factor	*All women*	*Menopausal status*	
		Pre	*Post*
Early age at menarche	1.5		
Late age at menopause			1.5
Early artificial menopause		0.4	
Nulliparity	2.5		
Late age at first birth	3.0		
Benign breast disease:			
No atypia	2.0		
With atypical hyperplasia	5.0		
High fat in the diet	1.5		
Family history of breast cancer	2.0	3.0	1.5
Lactation		0.5	1.0
Obesity		1.0	2.0
Use of oral contraceptives		1.0	
Use of non-contraceptive estrogens			1.5

Table 1 summarises the relative risks derived from a number of studies for the major risk factors for breast cancer. Some apply at all ages, some apply only to pre- or post-menopausal women. Early age at menarche (younger than 12), late age at menopause (older than 50), nulliparity and late age at first birth (older than 25 or particularly 30) which increase risk, and early artificial menopause (40 or younger) which reduces risk, are clearly related to hormone status. These are not necessarily independent. Thus, the protective effect of childbearing (most studies showing increasing protection with increasing number of children) seems to be largely explained by early age at first birth.

Other risk factors are not so obviously related to hormone status though some have postulated that the effect of diet may in part be mediated through a hormonal effect. For example, there is a clear relationship between improved nutrition and early age at menarche. Age at menarche has been falling in western countries, and is now falling in several developing countries and this could be a partial explanation for rising breast cancer incidence in many of them.

The remaining risk factors in the table vary according to a woman's menopausal status, and Chapter 2 discusses this for a family history of breast cancer. Lactation is commonly regarded as protective for breast cancer. Until a large international study in the 1960s, there were conflicting reports on this, but the study concluded that the critical risk factor was age at first birth, lactation having no independent effect in that study. However, two recent studies have suggested that lactation may indeed be protective for breast cancer in pre-menopausal women, but not in post-menopausal women. In contrast, obesity seems to increase the risk only in post-menopausal women and especially in women age 60 or more (see Chapter 6).

As breast cancer is often hormone dependent, it is perhaps surprising that the risk does not seem to be affected by the use of oral contraceptives (see Chapter 8). However, this finding applies only to the risk of breast cancer in pre-menopausal women, as women with prolonged intake of oral contraceptives are only now reaching their post-menopausal years. With regard to the use of estrogens for menopausal symptoms, there now seems to be consistent evidence for an increase in risk especially after prolonged use, and after 10 or more years from first use.

The Importance of Various Risk Factors: the Population Approach

Table 2 evaluates the importance of each risk factor in relation to the amount of breast cancer in the population *attributable* to the factor. Calculation of population-attributable risks requires knowledge of the proportion of people exposed to the factor as well as the relative risk. The proportion exposed may vary between populations but not all investigators publish this information. Therefore, there is more uncertainty about the estimates in Table 2 than for those in Table 1, and they are more likely to apply to a North American than to a European population. Nevertheless, they serve to place the risk factors in a different perspective from that examined in the first section.

In particular, obesity and high fat in the diet are seen to account for a substantial proportion of breast cancer in the population and this finding is perhaps welcome as these risk factors may be more readily modified than are family history or some of the hormonal risk factors. Although attributable risks in the population are not necessarily additive, recent evidence from Israel suggest that total fat intake and obesity contribute independently to increased risk. Given that the importance of diet may be underestimated because of the imprecision of current dietary estimates in epidemiology, it seems likely that diet and obesity might account for more than 50% of breast cancer in the population.

Table 2 Population attributable risk (PAR) for certain factors

Factor	*PAR %*
Early age at menarche	5–20*
Late age at menopause	10
Nulliparity	14
Late age at first birth	18
Benign breast disease	14
High fat in the diet	27
Family history of breast cancer	17
Lactation	(9)**
Obesity	12
Use of non-contraceptive estrogens	6

*Range given because some studies suggest effect may be restricted to pre-menopausal women (5% estimate).
**Protective effect.

Combining Risk Factors

If high dietary fat intake and obesity in the population approach can be regarded as contributing independently to the amount of breast cancer attributable to these factors in the population, is this true for the individual woman? There is very little guidance from the scientific literature on this question (except in regard to participation in screening programmes discussed in the next section) because the studies that were the basis for Tables 1 and 2 were generally concerned with the effect of risk factors separately. Cuzick *et al.* [1] have performed some theoretical estimates in identifying a high risk *group* of women, but their calculations cannot be applied to individual women.

There are some reasons, however, for believing that separate risk factors, if present in the same individual together, can 'interact', that is, multiply the effect of each other. DuPont and Page [2], for example, found that in women with atypical hyperplasia in a breast biopsy, the subsequent risk of breast cancer was five times that of women with non-proliferative lesions; but while a family history of breast cancer was associated with no increased risk to the individual with non-proliferative lesions, in those with atypical hyperplasia the effect of a family history of breast cancer was to increase the subsequent risk of breast cancer to 11 times that of a women with non-proliferative lesions and without a family history of breast cancer (see Chapter 5).

Although family history has been shown before to have such a multiplying effect on the risk caused by another factor, this cannot be assumed to apply universally. Some of the effects of diet, for example, may be mediated through early age at menarche, while it is possible that some of the effects of family history may be mediated through diet. Faced with an individual women, therefore, it is usual to consider the effect of risk factors on an individual basis. When doing so, it is important to bear in mind that risks are usually assessed by comparing those at highest risk with those at lowest. Thus in Table 1 an RR of 3 for late age at first birth is derived by comparing women whose first birth was later than 30 with women whose first birth was before 20. This does not mean that women whose first birth was over the age of 30 has three times the risk of an *average* woman, as the average includes those with early and late first births. Compared with an average women, a woman whose first birth was over the age of 30 is only at about 1.5 times increased risk.

Only rarely, therefore, is is justifiable to translate estimates of degree of risk into advice as extreme as a prophylactic bilateral mastectomy, and perhaps only then for those with the very rare genetically-dominant family history described by Lynch (see Chapter 3). A more reasonable approach is to adopt general preventive dietary manoeuvres that can also be recommended on general health grounds, such as lowering fat intake and maintaining ideal body weight, and (especially if over the age of 50) participating in screening programmes.

Thus, it would appear that on the basis of degree of risk there are limits to the counselling we can at present offer women regarding the primary or secondary prevention of breast cancer. At one extreme, the preventive manoeuvre of prophylactic mastectomy can be considered only in exceptionally rare instances. At the other extreme, general counselling regarding dietary modification and maintenance of ideal body weight should really be offered to *all* women on the basis of general health benefits. However, there is one currently available manoeuvre, namely screening, which can be offered to women on a discretionary basis. Attention has therefore turned to understanding the cumulative chance of a woman having a breast cancer detected by screening, so that women at high risk for breast cancer detection can be identified and counselled toward earlier and more frequent screening than those at low risk.

Selecting Woman for Participation in Screening Programmes

Only a few women can benefit from participation in screening programmes for breast cancer, other than from the assurance that at the time of the examination they do not have breast cancer. The only true beneficiaries are those who if they had developed breast cancer diagnosed in the normal way would have died from the disease, but when diagnosed following early detection in the screening programme, will receive effective treatment and will not die from breast cancer. If such women could be identified, it would be appropriate to concentrate screening on them.

Unfortunately, we are unable to identify these really high risk women (see Chapter 9) but we can increase the probability that those whom we label as high risk will include a greater proportion of the true beneficiaries of screening than those whom we label as low risk. We do this largely by using the available information in order to develop a formula which can discriminate between those at high and those at low risk.

There are many difficulties in this approach. First, we are using *diagnosis* of breast cancer as a surrogate for death from breast cancer, and yet we have seen that not all potential deaths from breast cancer are benefited by screening. Secondly, screening tends to identify a type of case that might not even have been diagnosed in the absence of screening thus leading to the problem of overdiagnosis by screening. If these cases form a high proportion of those considered in the analysis, then the answer we obtain on those who should be selected for screening may be totally irrelevant to those we should really like to screen.

Table 3 Results of discriminant analysis, symptoms excluded (Schechter *et al.* [5])

Approach	*Cancers detected*	*Healthy Screened*
Based on risk factor count		
One or more	94.4	85.9
Two or more	74.7	57.4
Three or more	45.7	24.2
Four or more	15.5	5.9
Five or more	2.8	0.8
Based on logistic model		
Critical value		
>−0.5	88.9	74.8
>−0.25	81.2	50.5
>0	77.7	39.7
>−0.25	58.3	28.8
>−0.5	30.6	9.3

Thirdly, as emphasised by Hakama, because our knowledge on risk factors for breast cancer is imperfect, selecting women to be screened will reduce the proportion of women who are not destined to develop cancer, but at the same time, some women who do develop it will not be screened. The more we attempt to concentrate on high risk women, the greater this effect will be. Thus, one early attempt to discriminate between women at high and low risk for breast cancer resulted in selecting 30% of women in the population to be screened, but only 40% of all women who developed breast cancer were thus selected [13]. A similar result has recently been reported from Edinburgh [4] where it was noted that if the aim was to screen only

20% of the healthy women, then only 30% of the total breast cancers would have been found. Even when the percentage of healthy women screened was increased to 48% only 56% of the total cancers were detected.

The Canadian National Breast Screening Study (NBSS) is setting up a randomised trial evaluating mammography and clinical examination of the breasts in nearly 90 000 women age 40–59 [5]. Table 3 shows the data derived from the initial screening examination of 30 718 women among whom 115 breast cancers were diagnosed. Using simple counts of the *number of risk factors* per woman gave only moderate discriminating power. By incorporating quantitative information on the *degree of risk* from the risk factors (discriminant analysis) it was possible to add to the discrimination provided by the other risk factors, and this was increased still further (particularly the presence of a lump) if information on symptoms was added.

The risk factors included in the analysis were age 50 or more, age 27 or more at first birth, nulliparity, positive family history of breast cancer, history of benign breast disease, age 12 or less at menarche (pre-menopausal women only), age 45 or more at menopause (post-menopausal women only), ever smoker (pre-menopausal women only), natural menopause (post-menopausal women only) and history of lumps, pain or discharge in preceding 6 months (when symptoms were included).

Just as we distinguished earlier between the individual-based and the population-based approach to risk factors, so too can selective screening be divided. A population-based selection strategy would rely entirely on epidemiologic risk factors, and only those women at sufficiently high risk based on some formulation of their known risk factors (such as family history, age at menarche, benign disease, age at first birth, etc.) would be invited. Current screening recommendations based on age and family or personal history represent a form of population-based selection.

Several attempts have been made to devise population-based selection strategies but with little success [3, 4, 6–9]. For example, Soini and Hakama [7] constructed a multivariate discriminant which correctly identified 85% of cases as being high risk but it also included the majority (65%) of healthy controls in this category. Alexander *et al.* [4] used 4 risk factors to define a high risk subgroup of 48% of women but it contained only 56% of all the cancers developing. Most would agree that the sensitivity of any selection should not fall below 80–90% otherwise the purpose of the screening could be nullified. However, in order to achieve this level of sensitivity, most population-level selection strategies to date have had to include the majority of healthy controls, nullifying to a marked degree the purpose of the selection.

Individually-based selection would appear to offer greater power of discrimination. Such selection processes can involve important factors such as symptomatology, clinical findings, and even previous mammographic results in the decision on whether or not to screen. Alexander *et al.* [4] proposed a theoretical strategy in which all women would be offered physical examination but only those with clinical findings and/or other risk factors would receive mammography. Their analysis revealed that such a selection would have detected 86% of all the first round cancers found in their programme using 52% of the mammographic resources. However, using only the information from the clinical examination, 69% of the cancers were detected with only 5% of the healthy given mammography. In the NBSS we found that multivariate selection incorporating symptoms, particularly the presence of a lump, would have detected 86% of the first screen cancers but would have screened only about 40% of the attendees.

Most research to date has addressed the question of the first screen and is not relevant to the issue of how frequently to screen once screening has begun. Effective decision rules might be designed to indicate the ideal frequency of screening for an individual woman based on her age, her risk profile, her clinical findings, and results from previous screens. This idea is currently under investigation within several screening programmes.

Risk Factors for Death from Breast Cancer

Few studies have evaluated the relationship of the above risk factors to survival from breast cancer. Newman *et al.* [10] studied the influence on breast cancer survival of age, weight and height at interview, age at first birth, and daily dietary intake of calories, total fat, saturated fat, oleic acid, linoleic acid and cholesterol. Only weight had a significant effect on breast cancer survival. The 5-year survival for those weighing 63 kg or more was 84% and that for those weighing less than 63 kg was 73%. This finding mirrored earlier clinical investigations that also showed an adverse effect of obesity on breast cancer survival [11, 12].

Conclusion

There are two perspectives from which risk factors for breast cancer can be viewed. The individual approach seeks to evaluate risk factors in terms of the risk they pose to the individual woman. The population approach seeks to evaluate risk factors in terms of how much disease in society can be attributed to that factor. The most important risk factors for breast cancer from the individual perspective are age, family history and ethnic origin. Other important risk factors are early menarche, nulliparity, late age at first birth, benign breast disease and high dietary fat, though these are not all independent. Other risk factors include late age at menopause, obesity, and possibly estrogen replacement therapy in post-menopausal women, while there may be a possible protective effect of lactation in pre-menopausal women.

Importance of a risk factor at the individual level does not necessarily imply importance at the population level. Thus, at the latter level, family history has less overall significance, while obesity and high fat in the diet could account for more than 50% of breast cancers.

Although there is some evidence that the effect of one risk factor may sometimes multiply the effect of another (e.g., family history and evidence of atypical hyperplasia in a biopsy) this cannot be assumed to apply generally. Risk for an individual should be considered in relation to average, not low, risk if extreme measures such as prophylactic mastectomy are contemplated.

Selective screening refers to the use of a selection rule to define a high-risk subgroup of women in whom screening is carried out. Differences observed in epidemiologic risk factors between detected cases and healthy screenees are not strong enough to permit population-level selection strategies. However, individually-based selection strategies, which incorporate symptoms and clinical findings into a selection index, may perform somewhat better.

References

1. Cuzick, J., Wang, D.Y., Bulbrook, R.D. (1986). The prevention of breast cancer. *Lancet*, **i**, 83–86.
2. DuPont, W.D., Page, D.L. (1985). Risk factors for breast cancer in women with proliferative breast disease. *New Engl. J. Med.*, **312**, 146–151.
3. Shapiro, S., Goldberg, J., Venet, L., Strax, P. (1973). Risk factors in breast cancer – a prospective study. In Doll, P. and Vodopija , I. (eds.), *Host Environment Interactions in the Etiology of Cancer in Man*, (IARC Scientific Publications no. 7), International Agency for Research on Cancer, Lyon, 169–182.
4. Alexander, F.E, Roberts, M.M., Huggins, A. (1987). Risk factors for breast cancer with applications for selection for the prevalance screen. *J. Epid. Comm. Hlth.*, **41**, 101–106.
5. Schechter, M.T., Miller, A.B., Baines, C.J., Howe, G.R. (1986). Selection of women at high risk of breast cancer for initial screening. *J. Chron. Dis.*, **39**, 253–260.
6. Farewell, V.T. (1977). The combined effect of breast cancer risk factors. *Cancer*, **40**, 931–936.
7. Soini, I., Hakama, M. (1978). Failure of selective screening for breast cancer by combining risk factors. *Int. J. Cancer*, **22**, 275–281.
8. de Waard, F., Rombach, J.J., Collette, H.J.A. (1978). The DOM-Project for the early diagnosis of breast cancer in the city of Utrecht, The Netherlands. In Miller, A.B. (ed.), *Screening for Cancer*, (UICC Technical Report Series, vol 40), International Union Against Cancer, Geneva, 183–200.
9. Toti, A., Piffanelli, A., Pacanelli, T. *et al.* (1980). Possible indication of breast cancer risk through discriminant function. *Cancer*, **46**, 1280–1285.
10. Newman, S.C., Miller, A.B., Howe, G.R. (1986). A study of the effect of weight and dietary fat on breast cancer survival time. *Amer. J. Epidem*, **123**, 767–774.
11. Boyd, N.F., Campbell, J.E., Germanson, T. *et al.* (1981). Body weight and prognosis in breast cancer. *J. Nat. Cancer Inst.*, **67**, 785–789.
12. Donegan, W.L., Hartz, A.J., Rimm, A.A. (1978). The association of body weight with recurrent cancer of the breast. *Cancer*, **41**, 1590–1594.

Chapter 8

Can Oral Contraceptives Reduce Breast Cancer Risk?

BASIL A. STOLL

The growing use of combined oral contraceptives (COC) in the Western world over the last 30 years, together with the increasing incidence of breast cancer [1] have led epidemiologists to search for a cause-and-effect relationship between the two trends. However, of the 10 or more large studies published in the last 10 years, most have found no evidence of an overall increased risk of breast cancer associated with the use of COC containing a mixture of oestrogen and progestogen. In spite of this, some clinicians are still wary because some of the studies have suggested a possible risk associated with prolonged use of the old type, high dose pill in younger women [2, 3].

This chapter will not only review the epidemiological evidence on the relationship, but also biological evidence that combining a progestogen with oestrogen is more likely to protect women against breast cancer than to promote it. One might expect reduction in breast cancer incidence from the use of COC also because of evidence that their use reduces the incidence of some types of benign breast disease and their administration as treatment can cause regression in established breast cancer.

There is a need for more epidemiological evidence as to the effect of COC consumption in different age and high-risk groups, and more biological evidence on the effect of different formulations and dosage of COC on the growth of breast tissue. It should then be possible to advise women on the timing and type of COC which might not only enable them to space their family but is likely at the same time to prevent or delay the appearance of breast cancer [4].

Epidemiological Evidence

Conflicting results have come from the various case control and cohort studies which have examined the relationship between the use of COC and subsequent development of breast cancer. The difficulties of interpretation are illustrated by the fact that two case control studies carried out by the same group at Oxford, UK, at different times came to opposite conclusions [5, 6]. The first indicated a moderate degree of protection conferred by taking COC, while the second found a threefold increased risk associated with 4 years use or more. A recent update of the second report [3] suggests that the increased risk is concentrated among women taking old type, high dose pills before their first full term pregnancy. Like the others, this study has been criticised on methodological grounds but in any case, these high dose pills have long been superseded in the UK.

Of the early studies relating the use of COC to breast cancer incidence, three showed no statistically significant change in risk from the use of the pill. While the first study [7] showed an overall non-significant reduction in risk, the second [8] showed a non-significant reduction in risk only among women aged 18–39, and the third study [9] showed a non-significant increase in risk among the COC users.

There were four early studies which did report a significantly increased risk of breast cancer among COC users but only in specific subgroups of women. In one study [1], use of COC by women without a family history of breast cancer was found to reduce their risk significantly, but if they had an aunt or grandmother with a history of breast cancer, they had a nearly five-fold increased risk for developing such a tumour. In another study, the risk was significantly increased in those women taking oral contraceptives for 2–4 years but not when they were taken for more than 4 years [11].

In the third study [12], there was no increased risk of breast cancer in women using the pill between the ages of 31–45 years, but its use between the ages of 46–55 led to an increased risk. The fourth study, which was given wide publicity at the time [2] claimed an increased risk of breast cancer in women under the age of 25 or in those with 4 or more years use of 'high-progestogen' pills. Since the progestogen potency of COC is difficult to quantify, the latter conclusion of this study has been refuted by most authorities, and in any case, the findings were not confirmed in the largest subsequent study [13].

Of the most recent studies, the largest in the USA [13] showed no significant change in risk regardless of duration of use, time since last use, use before first full term pregnancy or type of oestrogen or progestogen in the COC. A study from New Zealand [14] showed no overall increase in risk with over 10 years use of COC, but a Scandinavian report [15] showed a two-fold increase in risk with more than 12 years use of the pill.

Epidemiologists have focused on the effect of taking COC early in reproductive life, particularly in teenagers before the first pregnancy. Whereas some reports suggest an association between early use and increased risk in this group [2, 15–17], others disagree [13, 14, 18–20]. One report mentioned above suggests a doubled risk in younger women associated with the use of old type, high dose COC for a year or more before their first pregnancy [3].

There is now clear evidence that women taking COC have a *reduced* risk of developing endometrial or ovarian cancer. However, it must be taken into account that breast cancer (much more so than the other hormone-dependent cancers) represents the results of interaction between *several* genetic or life style factors, and changing only one of the multiple factors is likely to affect only *one sub-group* of women. Thus, one report suggested that COC increased breast cancer risk (but not significantly) in women with a maternal history of breast cancer but not in those with a history of benign breast disease [21]. Of the later studies, one suggested a higher incidence (again, not significant) in both groups [22] while three others found no evidence of increased risk in either of the groups [13, 19, 23]. One report suggested that the use of COC decreased the risk of breast cancer developing in women *without* a family history of disease (grandmother or aunt) but increased the risk in women *with* such a family history [10]. This applied particularly in premenopausal breast cancer.

It has been proposed that an association with risk of breast cancer might also vary according to the type of progestogen or oestrogen in the particular COC used. Thus, one report [2] claimed that those preparations with a high progestogenic potency were associated with an increased risk of breast cancer but not those with low potencies. These findings have not however been confirmed by others [20, 24]. Moreover, the progestogenic potency was based on effects on the uterine endometrium, not on the breast. With regard to the oestrogen component of the pill, one report [3] found that COC containing ethinyl oestradiol were associated with a higher risk of breast cancer than those containing the oestrogen mestranol. This seems unlikely on a biological basis because mestranol is rapidly converted in the body to ethinyl oestradiol following administration.

Because of the multiple factors involved in breast cancer development, the effect of COC on the risk of breast cancer may depend not only on its formulation but also on a woman's age at the time she first uses the agent, the duration and intermittency of administration, and its relationship in time to spontaneous changes in hormonal levels (such as pregnancy or miscarriage, the approach of the menopause or use of hormone replacement therapy). It may reduce the risk of breast cancer only in women without strong predisposing factors such as a family history of the disease or precancerous changes in the breast. The conflicting results of the epidemiological studies may be due to the difficulty of matching all risk factors in control groups, selection bias in the group examined, inadequate length of follow up or incomplete data concerning the formulation and dose of the various COC taken.

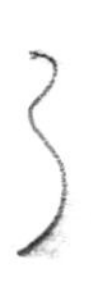

It has also been pointed out that if there was a protective effect from the use of COC it might be obscured by the fact that women using it are under closer medical surveillance than are non-users [25]. Thus, the apparent incidence of breast cancer among COC users may be inflated because a symptomless cancer is more likely to be discovered in such women. This suggestion is supported by the observation that in patients taking COC, less advanced tumours are found at the time of primary treatment [23].

To summarise this section: the populations considered in the epidemiological studies involve too many variable factors to provide comparable conclusions which can be applied to all women taking COC or to specific subgroups of women. Moreover, changes which are constantly occurring in the formulation of oral contraceptives mean that present findings relate to agents used 10–20 years ago, but have little relevance to the future incidence of breast cancer in COC users. Epidemiologists agree that it is too soon to expect significant relationships to emerge and that different combinations taken at different items in a woman's life may have quite different effects on her risk of developing breast cancer.

Evidence of Protective Effect by added Progestogen

Certain types of benign breast disease are widely accepted as being precancerous, particularly if they show microscopic evidence of epithelial atypia. Practically all studies examining this question agree that the use of COC is associated with a reduced risk of benign breast disease (for review see [26]). This is especially marked in women who have used the pill for more than two years, and it is claimed that eight or more years use leads to an 80% reduction in the incidence of benign breast disease. The protective effect of COC extends to both cystic disease and fibroadenoma of the breast but it is claimed in one report that the incidence of fibrocystic disease is reduced only if evidence or premalignant change is not already demonstrable in the ducts of the breast [27]. This finding is unconfirmed.

The unanimity of the observations relating the use of COC to a reduced incidence of benign breast disease contrasts with the conflicting findings relating it to the risk of breast cancer. It suggests that the formulation of COC in protecting against benign breast disease may not be as critical as it is for protecting against breast cancer. While most of the widely used COC contain both progestogen and oestrogen, the mechanism by which the pill reduces the incidence of benign breast disease is probably related to the progestogen component. Thus, an increased risk of fibrocystic disease has been noted among women taking oestrogen alone, and the greater the proportion of progestogen in the pill, the greater the protection from benign breast disease [28].

Clinical evidence of a protective effect of progestogen against breast cancer also is the observation that women with evidence of progesterone deficiency have a five-fold greater risk of developing breast cancer *before* the menopause, compared to those whose infertility is caused by other factors [29]. Another study showed that chronic failure to ovulate associated with progesterone deficiency increased the risk of breast cancer *after* the menopause by a factor of more than three [30]. Conversely, it appears that the administration of progestogen for a prolonged period is likely to decrease a woman's risk of breast cancer. Thus, a group of 246 women treated by 3-monthly depot injections of medroxyprogesterone for contraceptive purposes showed a reduced risk of breast cancer, although not to a statistically significant degree [31].

Further evidence of the protective effect of progestogen is provided by three studies showing that the addition of progestogen to oestrogen replacement therapy decreases the risk of developing breast cancer in postmenopausal women [32–34]. Those who did not receive hormone replacement therapy had a five-times greater incidence of breast cancer than those who received a progestogen/oestrogen formulation, while those who received oestrogen only, had an intermediate incidence [33].

In the case of established breast cancer also, treatment by progestogens counteracts the stimulating effect of oestrogen on the growth of chemically-induced breast cancer in animals [35] and also causes regression of human breast cancer both in pre- and post-menopausal women [36]. In the laboratory, the addition of progestogens can counteract the stimulating effect of oestrogen on the growth of human breast cancer cells [37]. With regard to combinations of oestrogen and progestogen, as in the pill, breast cancer in animals was inhibited by the COC Enovid [38] while the growth of established breast cancer in the human was inhibited by taking the COC Lyndiol at contraceptive dosage [39].

What is the relevance of observations of COC inhibition of established breast cancer to the possibility of cancer prevention by such COC? In the case of endometrial cancer, treatment by COC has been shown to cause regression of established cancer [40] while women taking COC show a reduced incidence of endometrial cancer [41]. In the case of breast cancer, we have noted above that the progestogen medroxyprogesterone can cause regression of established breast cancer [36] while the same agent used for contraceptive purposes can reduce the incidence of breast cancer [31]. There is then a basis for postulating that agents which cause regression of established cancer may also reduce the risk of developing the disease. Most important, it could provide a way to select a particular COC which may be more suitable for use by women at high risk to breast cancer.

The mechanism involved in reducing the incidence of breast cancer by COC might either be by delaying promotion changes or by reversing premalignant changes (see Chapter 1). There is also a suggestion that, in women taking COC, the growth rate of subsequently appearing breast cancer may be slowed, as shown by reports that such tumours in COC users may be less aggressive than in non-users. A British study [42] noted a 5 year survival rate of 96% in patients with breast cancer developing in pill users compared to 78% in non-users, and 10 year survival rates of 74% and 46% respectively. A similar inquiry in the USA [24] found that 55% of non-users had died of the disease but only to 42% of those women using COC when breast cancer was diagnosed. On the other hand, a recent report has found neither increase nor decrease in the extent of the disease at presentation, nor improvement in survival rates, in women taking COC [43].

Where do We Go from Here?

It is widely agreed that the disparate results relating the use of the pill to breast cancer incidence are due in part to the considerable variation throughout the world in the formulation of the different oral contraceptives used since their general introduction over 30 years ago. The biological effect of these agents depends critically on the formulation [44]. It might therefore be more profitable to direct more research into the biological effects of various oestrogen/progestogen combinations upon the growth of human breast epithelium and breast cancer, and to try to distinguish the relative roles of oestrogen and progestogen in growth and differentiation control. Using human breast cancer cell lines in the laboratory, oestrogen at moderate dose levels is most often growth stimulating but at high doses almost universally inhibiting [45]. Progesterone alone usually has no effect on the growth of such cell lines but a moderate dose level may in some cases be stimulating while in others it is inhibiting.

Few attempts have been made to compare the effect of different COC and their constituent oestrogens and progestogens on the growth of normal and malignant cells from the human breast in the laboratory. One such attempt noted stimulation in about 75% of the malignant specimens by progestogens or COC, but this did not apply to the normal breast tissue [46]. The agents showed considerable variation in their stimulating ability but equivalent concentrations of the various progestogens were used and no allowance was made for the very different potencies of the agents. Differences could also be partly explained by differences in the degree to which various progestogens are converted into their active metabolites under laboratory conditions. Any attempt to extrapolate laboratory data to the clinic must take such factors into account.

Nevertheless, it was observed [46] that (a) malignant cells responded differently from normal cells to the same agent; (b) malignant cells from different women responded differently to the same agent. Differences in response may be due either to variations in the enzyme systems necessary to activate an agent, or to differences in the level of steroid receptors in the cells. Further studies need to be carried out to investigate the effect of the agents at a concentration which more closely resembles that found clinically.

What is the significance of a growth-stimulating effect by progestogens on breast cancer cells in the laboratory when these agents are being widely used to cause regression in advanced breast cancer? In the patient, the need for oestrogen priming before progestogen therapy is suggested by the observation that regression of breast cancer is much more likely in postmenopausal cases if they show evidence of persistent oestrogen secretion [47]. In addition, a combination of progestogen and oestrogen (as in the COC Lyndiol) has been shown to cause a higher regression rate in postmenopausal patients with advanced breast cancer [39].

To summarise this section: in the body, COC are likely to inhibit the proliferative activity of human breast cancer cells but the degree may depend on the formulation of the agent, its metabolism in the body, its circulating level in the blood and its uptake by the cancer cells. On the basis of available evidence, it is more likely to be beneficial than harmful to prescribe either a combination-type hormone replacement therapy (oestrogen plus progestogen) or low dose COC, for patients with a history of breast cancer who are suffering from severe menopausal symptoms [48]. Similar advice can be given for the management of such symptoms in women with a family history of breast cancer.

There is now considerable biological evidence to support the hypothesis that while oestrogen stimulates breast cell growth, progestogen is likely to inhibit it. That progestogen stimulates differentiation and maturation in oestrogen-primed cells has been shown in the laboratory for both normal and malignant human breast cells (for review see [49]). Thus, progestogens are likely to reduce breast cancer risk by diverting the cells from proliferation to differentiation.

With regard to the effect of COC on breast cancer risk in normal women, the effect of COC must depend critically on their formulation, total duration and intermittency of their usage, the age when they were started in relation to the onset of menstruation, and their subsequent timing in relation to pregnancies, miscarriages and the approach of the menopause. The number of possible variations is enormous, and militates against recognising specific subgroups of women who show either adverse or beneficial effects on breast cancer risk. It may be possible that in the next 10–20 years a clear picture will emerge on the relationship between the use of COC and risk of developing breast cancer. The use of COC among young women did not become widespread until about 20 years ago and most breast cancers do not manifest until after the age of 40. It is likely that by the time we have amassed more conclusive results, vastly different formulations will be in use and findings will have little relevance to the cancer risk of current COC users.

New developments in contraception are increasingly using progestogen-only formulations. Vaginal rings or intrauterine devices, which release the progestogen levonorgestrel slowly, have been under trials for some years. The former device has to be replaced after 3 months and the latter after about 5 years. Their advantages are that, apart from having to rely less on the patient's memory, the side effects of the agent are less because of the local absorption of the progestogen. In addition to increasing use of these new progestogen-only agents, antiprogesterone agents are now available as morning-after pills. Finally, depot preparations of the hypothalamic hormone LHRH show promise of being safe and effective alternatives to COC when implanted as depots under the skin.

What advice can be given on COC usage to women at high risk for breast cancer? The evidence suggests that a combination of oestrogen and progestogen in specific doses and ratio may protect a woman against breast cancer if used at a critical time in her reproductive life. Laboratory and clinical research need to be carried out urgently to establish these critical factors. We need experimental models in which transplanted breast tissue and cancer can be induced to grow and differentiate under the influence of oestrogen in combination with progestogen, in order to mimic changes occurring in pregnancy. The use of explants into thymectomised mice has been suggested for the purpose [50].

Conclusion

Epidemiological observations are conflicting but there is no clear evidence that the use of oral contraceptives increases the overall risk of developing breast cancer. It is likely that the confusion is due to the numerous formulations of the pill which have been used for different durations at different times in their reproductive lives, by women who differ in their hereditary predisposition, production of natural steroids and metabolism of administered hormones. In looking for a major effect on breast cancer risk, we are looking for an effect on promotion and we may have to wait for another 10–15 years before we can expect more conclusive evidence.

Research needs to be devoted more to the effect of various synthetic progestogens in counteracting oestrogen support of breast cancer growth. There is considerable biological evidence which suggests that certain formulations of the pill can reduce the risk of breast cancer in both premenopausal and postmenopausal women as well as provide an effective method of birth control. Biological research on suitable models is essential if we are to identify these formulations.

References

1. Bailar, J.C., Smith, E.M. (1986). Progress against cancer? *New Engl. J. Med.*, **314**, 1226–1232.
2. Pike, M.C., Henderson, B.E., Krailo, M.D. *et al.* (1983). Breast cancer in young women and use of oral contraceptives. Possible modifying effect of formulation and age at use. *Lancet*, **ii**, 926–930.

3. McPherson, K., Vessey, M.P., Neil, A. *et al.* (1987). Early oral contraceptive use and breast cancer. *Brit. J. Cancer*, **56**, 653–660.
4. Scott, J.S. (1987). Oral contraceptives and breast cancer. *Lancet*, **ii**, 1526.
5. Vessey, M.P., McPherson, K., Yeates, D. *et al.* (1982). Oral contraceptive use and abortion before first pregnancy in relation to breast cancer risk. *Brit. J. Cancer*, **45**, 322–331.
6. McPherson, K., Neil, A., Vessey, M.P., Doll, R. (1983). Oral contraceptives and breast cancer. *Lancet*, **ii**, 1414–1415.
7. National Cancer Institute (1980). *Surveillance, Epidemiology and End Results (SEER)*, Biometry Branch of the National Cancer Institue, Bethesda, Md, 47.
8. Ramcharan, S., Pellegrin, F.A., Ray, R. *et al.* (1981). *The Walnut Creek Contraceptive Drug Study: a prospective study of the side effects of oral contraceptives*, vol. 3, DHHS (NIH), Bethesda, Md.
9. Kay, C. (1981). Breast cancer and oral contraceptives: findings in Royal College of General Practitioner's Study. *Brit. Med. J.*, **282**, 2089–2994.
10. Black, M.M., Barclay, T.H.C., Polednak, A. *et al.* (1983). Family history, oral contraceptive usage and breast cancer. *Cancer*, **51**, 2147–2151.
11. Fasal, E., Paffenbarger, R.S. Jr (1975). Oral contraceptives as related to cancer and benign lesions of the breast. *J. Nat. Cancer Inst.*, **55**, 757–762.
12. Jick, H., Walker, A.M., Watkins, R.N. *et al.* (1980). Oral contraceptives and breast cancer. *Amer. J. Epidem.*, **112**, 577–584.
13. Cancer and Steroid Hormone Study (1986). Oral contraceptive use and the risk of breast cancer. *N. Engl. J. Med.*, **315**, 405–411.
14. Paul, C., Skegg, D.C.G., Spears, G.F.S., Kaldor, K.M. (1986). Oral contraceptives and breast cancer; a national study. *Brit. Med. J.*, **293**, 723–726.
15. Meirik, O., Adami, H.O., Christofferson, T. *et al.* (1986). Oral contraceptive use and breast cancer in young women. *Lancet*, **ii**, 650–653.
16. Paffenbarger, R.S., Fasal, E., Simmons, M.E. *et al.* (1977). Cancer risk as related to oral contraceptives during fertile years. *Cancer*, **39**, 1887–1891.
17. Olsson, H., Olsson, M., Muller, T.R. *et al.* (1985). Oral contraceptive use and breast cancer in young women in Sweden. *Lancet*, **i**, 748–749.
18. Janerich, D.T., Poldnak, A.P., Glebatis, D.M., Lawrence, C.E. (1983). Breast cancer and oral contraceptive use; a case control study. *J. Chron. Dis.*, **36**, 639–646.
19. Rosenberg, L., Miller, D.R., Kaufman, D.W. *et al.* (1984). Breast cancer and oral contraceptive use. *Amer. J. Epidem.*, **119**, 167–176.
20. Stadel, B.V., Rubin, G.L., Webster, L.A. *et al.* (1985). Oral contraceptives and breast cancer in young women. *Lancet*, **ii**, 970–971.
21. Paffenbarger, R.S., Kampert, J.B., Chang, H.G. (1979). Oral contraceptives and breast cancer risk. *INSERM*, **83**, 93–114.
22. Brinton, L.A., Hoover, R., Szklo, M., Fraumeni, J.F. (1982). Oral contraceptives and breast cancer. *Int. J. Epidem.*, **11**, 316–322.
23. Vessey, M., Baron, J., Doll, R. *et al.* (1983). Oral contraceptives and breast cancer; final report of an epidemiological study. *Brit. J. Cancer*, **47**, 455–462.
24. Gambrell, R.D. Jr (1984). Oral contraceptives, postmenopausal oestrogen-progestogen use and breast cancer. *J. Obstet. Gynecol.*, **4**, s? 121–126.
25. Realini, J.P. (1987). Oral contraceptive use and the risk of breast cancer. *New Engl. J. Med.*, **316**, 163.
26. Fentiman, I.S., Wang, D.Y. (1986). Hormonal background of benign breast disease. *Rev. Endoc. Related Cancer*, **24**, 11–16.
27. LiVolsi, V.A., Stadel, B.V., Kelsey, J.L. *et al.* (1978). Fibrocystic breast disease in oral contraceptive users. *N. Engl. J. Med.*, **299**, 381–385.

28. Royal College of General Practitioners (1977). Effect on hypertension and benign breast disease of progestogen component in combined oral contraceptives. *Lancet*, **i**, 624–626.
29. Cowan, O.D., Gordis, L., Tonascia, J.A. *et al.* (1981). Breast cancer incidence in women with a history of progesterone deficiency. *Amer. J. Epidem.*, **114**, 209–213.
30. Coulan, C.B., Annergers, J.F. (1983). Chronic anovulation may increase postmenopausal breast cancer risk. *J. Amer. Med. Ass.*, **249**, 445–447.
31. WHO Collaborative Study (1984). Breast cancer, cervical cancer and depot medroxyprogesterone acetate. *Lancet*, **i**, 1207–1208.
32. Nachtigall, L.E., Nachtigall, R.H., Nachtigall, R.D. *et al.* (1979). Estrogen replacement, II. A prospective study in the relationship to carcinoma and cardiovascular and metabolic problems. *Obstet. Gynecol.*, **54**, 74–76.
33. Gambrell, R.D. Jr, Maier, R.C., Sanders, B.I. (1983). Decreased incidence of breast cancer in postmenopausal estrogen-progestogen users. *Obstet. Gynecol.*, **62**, 435–438.
34. Lauritzen, C., Meier, F. (1984). Risks of endometrial and mammary cancer morbidity and mortality in long-term oestrogen treatment. In Herendael, H. and B., Ripwagen, F.E., Goessens, I., van der Pas, H. (eds.), *The Climacteric – An Update*, MTP Press, Lancaster, 207–216.
35. Huggins, C., Yang, N.C. (1962). Induction and extinction of mammary cancer. *Science*, **137**, 257–262.
36. Buzdar, A.U. (1988). Progestins in cancer treatment. In Stoll, B.A. (ed.), *Contemporary Endocrine Therapy in Cancer*, S. Karger, Basel, 1–15.
37. Allegra, J.C., Kiefer, S.M. (1985). Mechanisms of action of progestational agents. *Semin. Oncol.*, **12**, (Suppl. 1), 3–5.
38. Welsch, C.W., Meites, J. (1969). Effects of Enovid on development and growth of carcinogen-induced mammary tumors in female rats. *Cancer*, **23**, 601–607.
39. Stoll, B.A. (1967). Effect of Lyndiol, an oral contraceptive, on breast cancer. *Brit. Med. J.*, **7**, 150–153.
40. Stoll, B.A. (1961). A new progestational steroid in the therapy of endometrial carcinoma. *Cancer Chemother. Rep.*, **14**, 83–84.
41. Gambrell, R.D. (1988). Hormonal medication and mitogenic dangers. In Stoll, B.A. (ed.), *Contemporary Endocrine Therapy in Cancer*, S. Karger, Basel, 126–143.
42. Matthews, P.N., Mills, P.R., Hayward, J.L. (1981). Breast cancer in women who have taken contraceptive steroids. *Brit. Med. J.*, **282**, 774–776.
43. Rosner, D., Lane, W.W., Brett, R.P. (1985). Influence of oral contraceptives on the prognosis of breast cancer in young women. *Cancer*, **55**, 1556–1562.
44. Anderson, T.J. (1984). Mitotic and apoptotic response of breast tissue to oral contraceptives. *Lancet*, **i**, 99–100.
45. Welsch, C.W. (1988). Personal communication.
46. Longman, S.M., Buehring, G.C. (1987). Oral contraceptives and breast cancer; *In vitro* effect of contraceptive steroids on human mammary cell growth. *Cancer*, **59**, 281–287.
47. Stoll, B.A. (1967). Vaginal cytology as an aid to hormone therapy in postmenopausal breast cancer. *Cancer*, **20**, 1807–1811.
48. Stoll, B.A., Parbhoo, S. (1988). Treatment of menopausal symptoms in breast cancer patients. *Lancet*, **i**, 1278–1279.
49. Gompel, A., Malet, C., Spritzen, P. *et al.* (1986). Progestin effect on cell proliferation and 17β-hydrogenase activity in normal human breast cells in culture. *J. Clin. Endocrin. Metab.*, **63**, 1174-1180.
50. McManus, M.J., Welsch, C.W. (1984). The effect of estrogen, progesterone, thyroxine and HPL on DNA synthesis of human breast ductal epithelium maintained in athymic nude mice. *Cancer*, **54**, 1920–1927.

Chapter 9

Clinical Cost–Benefit of Screening Programmes

RUTH ELLMAN

Breast cancer screening trials have provided the first clear evidence that early treatment can prolong life. The trials, in order to provide valid evidence on whether life is prolonged, have been based on comparisons of mortality from breast cancer in defined populations followed over several years. Results from two such population-based trials of breast cancer screening (one in New York, the HIP study [1], the other in Sweden, the Two Counties study [2] have, so far, been published and both show a 30% reduction in breast cancer mortality attributable to screening.

Studies which are limited to comparing the survival of screen-detected and otherwise-detected cases suffer from serious biases of which lead-time bias is the most important: earlier treatment as a result of screening prolongs survival even when treatment is ineffectual simply because survival is measured from the date of treatment.

Case-control studies comparing the screening histories of women who have died of breast cancer and women living in the same area who have not, have been devised to avoid lead-time bias but suffer from the possibility of a self-selection bias: women who have worrying breast symptoms may avoid screening for fear of diagnosis of cancer. Such a bias is evident in the higher detection rate observed in non-attenders in the Swedish trial. Nevertheless, the findings from case-control studies from Holland [3, 4] and Italy [5], which suggest that the risk of death from breast cancer in women who have attended screening is about 50% lower than in those who did not, add support to the findings of the two population-based studies, as does the consistency of indirect evidence from several other contemporary studies.

The main benefit of screening is prolonged life but another anticipated benefit is less costly and less unpleasant treatment. At present, treatment for early stage cancer is not necessarily more conservative. In six health districts which were not providing mammographic screening but were observed within the UK Trial of Early Detection of Breast Cancer from 1980–86, the proportion of Stage I cancers treated by mastectomy (as opposed to lumpectomy) varied from 51% to 82% and use of chemotherapy from 0% to 16%.

Predicting the Effects of Mass Screening

It is impossible yet to estimate with any accuracy the long-term benefit from a mass screening programme. First, because trials have not been continued for long enough. The New York trial used mammography which was primitive by present-day standards and only provided four annual screens, though the populations have been followed for 18 years; the Swedish Two Counties study has, as yet, published results based on mean follow-up of only 7 years. For a disease with a mean survival of about this length, the follow-up is insufficient to tell what effect screening has on the more slowly progressive cancers and whether the observed reduction in deaths indicates cure or only delay in recurrence.

Secondly, there is uncertainty because of the size of studies. Though the Swedish trial involved 163 000 women, results so far published [6] are based on only 197 breast cancer deaths, and the 32% reduction in mortality for women first screened between the ages of 40 and 74 has a 95% confidence interval of 10–45%.

Thirdly, forecasting from the Two Counties trials, the expertise and dedication of the research team must be taken into account. The recruitment and training of competent staff, the effective management of quality control systems, public education and service responsiveness to criticism, are all important in achieving a high screening acceptance rate and maximum benefit. Mere provision of access to screening is not enough. Breast cancer screening by gynaecologists has been encouraged in West Germany through a free voucher system since 1971 but has had no detectable effect on breast cancer mortality, nor has there been a fall in mortality in the USA, where, for over a decade, mammographic screening has been publicly encouraged but not financed and little controlled.

Decisions cannot wait for certainty but must make the best use of available information. The recent UK decision to introduce 3-yearly mammographic screening for women between the ages of 50 and 64 years, was based on the mortality experience of the Swedish trial during its first 7 years and on the longer term follow-up of the New York trials. It led to an estimate that such a programme would save 11.5 years of life over a period of 15 years for a cohort of 1000 women invited to screening [7]. More accurate estimates must await longer follow-up of the Swedish trial, by the addition of information from other population-based studies such as those in the UK, Holland, Italy, Canada and elsewhere in Sweden, and the experience of mass screening programmes themselves.

Evidence of Screening Benefit for Different Age Groups

The UK decision to invite only women over 50 years for screening was based on the failure of trials so far to demonstrate a definite reduction in mortality for younger women. Small cancers in pre-menopausal women are more difficult to detect because the breast tissue is less compressible and appears more dense of the mammogram. Possibly the initial growth rate is also accelerated in younger women.

Despite the lack of evidence, it is reasonable to hope that screening women under 50 years could prevent some deaths both before and after 50 , and it is argued that young women should be screened more frequently and with greater intensity than older women [8]. However, judgement on this issue must take into account the known disadvantages of screening as well as the potential benefits [9]. Among older women, screening trials have found a lower response to invitation, perhaps reflecting a perception that, as one grows older, screening offers less potential benefit in years of healthy life saved.

Alternative Methods of Screening

Clinical Examination

Screening in the New York study was both clinical and mammographic. At that time the sensitivity of mammographic screening was inferior to that of clinical examination. By the late 1970s mammography has greatly improved and the Swedish Two Counties study not only relied on single-view mammography alone but also extended the interval between screenings. The screening interval in the New York study was 12 months, in the Swedish study it varied from two to three years.

When used in conjunction with mammography, clinical examination adds 5–20% to the number of cancers detected. Some of the extra cases, however, are in women with symptoms. A simple questionnaire and a note by the radiographer of any visible deformity may help pick up these cases without resorting to full clinical examination of all women screened. In North America, however, clinical examination is considered an essential part of every screening [10].

Comparison of the sensitivity of two screening techniques used simultaneously may not predict the true contribution each makes to prolonging lives, but the expense of population-based mortality studies comparing different techniques is prohibitive. A Canadian trial [11] in which volunteers have been randomly allocated either to receive clinical screening alone or to receive mammographic plus clinical screening, is unique in attempting a rigorous comparison of the costs and benefits of two methods. It is to be hoped that well-monitored screening services, though not primarily intended for research, will also eventually yield evidence on the relative benefits of the different screening methods they adopt.

Breast Self-Examination (BSE)

Breast cancers reported to have been picked up as a result of routine self-examination tend to be smaller than those picked up by chance [12], but reporting is subject to bias. The UK Trial of Early Detection of Breast Cancer is the only trial in which the effect of this form of screening on population-based breast cancer mortality has been studied, though trials have recently been mounted in Leningrad. Results of the UK trial for the first 7 years have shown no mortality reduction attributable to the BSE programmes. Proponents of BSE may attribute this apparent failure to the low attendance (51% and 37% in the two BSE centres respectively), and to the fact that group education on only one occasion was given, rather than repeated individual practical demonstration.

On theoretical grounds, examination of a woman's breasts at monthly intervals must be capable of detecting signs earlier than yearly clinical screening. However, objectivity in self-assessment is difficult and may be especially so when the reward for discovery is an unpleasant one [13]. Even though a high proportion of women can be persuaded to try BSE, some give up, disconcerted by the lumpiness they observe but cannot accurately remember for later comparison. Others practise BSE regularly, but when they discover a suspicious change tend to panic, disbelieve the evidence for fear of being thought neurotic and so delay seeking treatment. Thus psycho-social factors and not simply technical competence may determine the success of BSE.

Delay in seeking treatment is still common in Britain, and perhaps contributes to Britain's high breast cancer mortality rate. Education which emphasizes to women the importance of prompt reporting of breast changes other than premenstrual ones, and to doctors the importance of adequate and sympathetic investigation, may be more valuable than concentration on BSE technique. As an adjunct to mammographic screening, BSE may help women to cope with the knowledge that mammographic screening is not fully effective and it may be performed more confidently once screening has established a baseline of normality.

Miscellaneous Techniques

Other techniques which have been compared with mammography are thermography, ultrasonography, transillumination and nuclear magnetic resonance imaging. Thermography which relies on the detection of warmth generated by the increased vascularity of some tumours is attractive in that it involves no prodding or X-rays: bras containing colourful thermosensitive liquid crystals could be sold to women for self-diagnosis. However, the very poor sensitivity and specificity of thermography when used to detect small cancers renders it worthless for mass screening and most inappropriate for self-screening. Transillumination methods, using visible or infra-red rays, suffer from a similar lack of sensitivity and specificity, but are being further developed.

Ultrasound has an established value in the differential diagnosis of localised solid tumours and cysts. For screening, however, it is necessary to scan the whole breast, area by area, and this makes ultrasonography a more expensive method than mammography, even if automated equipment is used. It is also less sensitive: when tested on a series of 1000 women it picked up only 58% of 64 cancers which were detected by mammography and only 8% of those under one centimetre [14]. Micro-calcification, which is often a marker of *in situ* cancer, is not detectable by ultrasound. Nuclear magnetic resonance imaging is likewise too expensive to be considered seriously for screening and also fails to detect micro-calcification.

Mammographic Screening

Mammography is still in the phase of rapid development and managers are faced with many choices concerning equipment and organization. In Britain, the mass screening programme is intended initially to copy the Swedish achievement of a 30–40% reduction in mortality from breast cancer among invited women at minimal cost; programmes seeking to provide more intensive and costly screening will only be encouraged where they serve a research purpose. The Swedish government, on the other hand, has accepted the argument for more intensive screening on the basis that it will reduce the incidence of cases occurring with symptoms in the intervals between screenings. They have not waited for proof that this will result in a greater reduction in mortality.

General purpose radiographic machines are not suitable for screening. Dedicated equipment with rare earth target tubes and screen-film combinations is essential. Grids improve picture quality but at the expense of greater irradiation. Even with good equipment the image can be marred by technical faults and poor film developing, so that regular quality checks are essential. Image quality is also dependent on the degree of compression of the breast and on accurate assessment of the exposure needed for the thickness of breast to be filmed.

Single-view screening was used in the Swedish study, but two views are more informative. The extra cost has to be balanced against the benefit of seeing lesions which may be off-side on the first film, obscured by structures such as the nipple or difficult to interpret without three-dimensional information. Careful positioning of the breast in single-view mammography can reduce the need for a second view, but two-view screening may prove cost-effective in some programmes (especially at a first screening) if it substantially lowers the proportion of women who need to be recalled for further investigations. Direct comparison of the sensitivity, staff-time involvement and recall rates using one and two-view mammography is needed.

Few people are at present trained in reading screening mammograms. Even radiologists with experience of conventional mammography require several months to become expert. It demands skill, yet the low probability of finding a cancer on screening films makes the job of routine screening unattractive to many radiologists. They may consider delegating the routine reading of films to other carefully selected and trained staff, but must set a low threshold for referring films and must themselves have extensive experience in screening. Otherwise, large numbers of biopsies and/or a low cancer detection rate will result. Employment of lower salaried staff is not cost-effective if sensitivity and specificity fall [15]. Double reading of films (as practised in the Swedish Two County study) reduces the chance of missing cancers but, again, increases the cost.

The UK programme proposes three-yearly screening for women over 50, Sweden 2-yearly screening, whilst the United States recommendations are for annual screening. Fewer cases of advanced cancer will undoubtedly occur if screening frequency is increased but the effect of such changes on mortality cannot be accurately predicted. Demand for frequent screening should not divert attention from the need to achieve a high coverage of the target population. The Swedish Two Counties study obtained the initial compliance of 90% of invited women and other research programmes have persuaded 60–80% of women to attend, whilst screening in the USA has only attracted a minority of women to participate.

The importance of wide coverage is well illustrated by the success of cervical screening programmes in reducing cervical cancer mortality in those Nordic countries (Sweden, Iceland and parts of Denmark) which achieved high levels of attendance through individual invitation [16]. This is in contrast to the hardly discernible impact of programmes in Britain which adopted a *laissez-faire* attitude.

Disadvantages of Screening

The disadvantages of screening have to be viewed from the point of view of the individual, of the health service and of society in general. Financial costs to the health service are the easiest to quantify.

Costs to the Health Service

Cost estimates for a single screening test vary according to assumptions made about apportionment of overheads, capital depreciation on equipment and on factors which are accidental or can be varied, such as throughput. Nevertheless, estimates from Sweden, Britain and Holland are reasonably similar with the average cost of a single view mammographic screen, including subsequent outpatient investigations ranging from £10 to £15 at 1984 prices. In the USA, where no screening is publicly financed, the cost, exclusive of further investigations, averages $80 but varies very widely.

In judging the value of a screening programme, cost per quality-adjusted year of life saved (QALYS) is the ideal measure, but life *quality* measurement has not yet been attempted. The Forrest Committee [7] arrived at a figure of £3000 per year of life saved by 3-yearly mammography, but since precise information on years of life saved by modern mammographic screening is lacking, the estimate is a very rough one. Others have produced more optimistic cost assessments or even suggested that breast cancer screening might reduce health service costs: such calculations have failed to discount future costs or have made the assumption that women cured of breast cancer remain healthy and independent until death.

The cost per case detected has the advantage of being more directly measurable and is useful when comparing different programmes, provided like is compared with like. Cost per case detected at first screening is lower than at later screenings because the prevalence of screen detectable cases is higher; the cost per case is also lower the older the women screened, and in self-invited women the cost per screen-detected case may appear unusually favourable due to inclusion of women with early symptoms or with a strong family history of breast cancer. In this rapidly developing field, economic modelling will be needed to predict the effect on cost per case detected of changes, such as alteration in disease prevalence, in throughput, in recall rates or in the type of further investigation as well as changes due to simple alterations in unit costs.

A mass screening programme requires, in addition to money, an expansion of health service staff and specialized training programmes. The extra staff required for a screening programme to cover five million women in the UK is estimated (in full-time equivalents) to be over 900 [7]. This includes almost 50 radiologists and 200 radiographers and also small increases in histopathology and surgical staffing, to cope with extra biopsies and the problems involved in localizing non-palpable breast lesions. The demand for assessments and treatments is particularly high during the start-up phase of screening and is one of the factors determining the rate at which screening enrolment can proceed.

Selective Screening and Cost-Effectiveness

Fifteen to thirty per cent of cancers occur in women who have none of the recognised risk factors for breast cancers (other than their sex, age and country of domicile). It is therefore not appropriate to exclude any women from screening (see Chapter 7) but it may be feasible to increase cost-effectiveness by using a questionnaire and the findings at previous screenings to assess risk and vary the screening interval accordingly [17].

The selective inclusion of high risk younger women is contentious, not only because the cost per case detected will be high due to the lower sensitivity and specificity of screening in young women, but especially because the benefits remain unproven. Emotional argument, that it is better to do something than wait passively, may prevail but the likely disadvantages and benefits as they apply to each individual must be compared with those of other strategies such as regular self-examination, non-radiographic screening or prophylactic mastectomy.

Radiation-Induced Cancer

The realization that mammography might actually cause cancer provoked a sudden fall in demand for screening in the USA in 1976. Careful review of the evidence, however, is reassuring [18]. Evidence comes principally from the long-term follow-up of Japanese women exposed to atom-bomb fall-out and of women subjected to repeated fluoroscopy during tuberculosis treatment. Exposure to ionizing radiation causes breast cancer but the effect is delayed for over 10 years. Exposure to 10 mGy (1 rad), which is the dose from a series of five mammograms, in a population of a million 50-year-old women would eventually causes about 50 extra breast cancer deaths, but the women would suffer five to ten thousand fewer breast cancer deaths on account of early treatment of disease detected by the screening. Benefit far outweighs risk, but nevertheless the risk must be kept to a minimum by regular checking of mammographic equipment and control of the number of radiographic exposures that women receive.

In younger women no benefit has yet been found to counterweight the risk, and indeed the risk is slightly increased since more exposure is often required to obtain good pictures. An added concern, based on the theory that cancer results from a series of genetic mutations, some of which can be inherited, is that women with a familial predisposition to breast cancer may be especially susceptible to the carcinogenic effect of irradiation.

The Increase in Operations Resulting from Screening

In the UK, in the absence of screening, the ratio of benign to malignant biopsies is lightly less than one to one in women over 50 years. Experienced screening teams in Sweden, Holland and UK keep the ratio below 2:1, but in earlier screening programmes much higher biopsy rates occurred. In North America, where biopsy rates are generally higher (and mastectomy rates are twice as high as in Britain), a benign to malignant ratio of 8:1 has been defended as necessary to the success of screening in younger women [19].

Costs of excessive biopsies are not simply financial. Biopsies are usually conducted under general anaesthesia and carry a risk of post-operative mortality (albeit very small), in addition to the more common problems of delayed healing, scar pain and breast disfigurement.

Overdiagnosis

The possibility of overdiagnosis is evident from the prevalence of occult breast cancer discovered by meticulous examination of breasts at autopsy. Nielsen [20] studied breast tissue at autopsy in a consecutive series of 110 women aged 20–54 years examined for medico-legal reasons. The prevalence was 20%, whereas the cumulative lifetime risk of developing breast cancer in Denmark is only 6.5%. Eleven percent of these cancers were detectable on specimen radiography. Nielsen also found a high prevalence (19%) in autopsies on elderly women. The more sensitive mammography becomes, the greater the risk that cancers which would not have caused symptoms during a woman's lifetime will be diagnosed and treated. This risk can be further increased by erroneous pathological reporting.

Overdiagnosis did not occur in the New York study but in the Swedish Two Counties study seven years after commencement there was still a 30% excess of invasive breast cancer. The excess could be due to long lead times, but overdiagnosis is also a possibility. Whether overdiagnosis is acceptable as a disadvantage of screening will depend on the extent to which the quality of life is reduced following treatment for early breast cancer. Once again, it is in younger women that the dilemma is greatest. Treatment trials have found that chemotherapy increases the proportion of premenopausal women with early stage cancer who survive 10 years by about 15% but views differ on whether a survival benefit for a small minority justifies the morbidity caused by the treatment.

Psychological Costs for Non-cancer patients

Opposition to screening arises in part from concern that increased medicalization of society is itself unhealthy [21]. Invitation to screening may arouse fear of cancer, fear of embarrassment or discomfort at mammographic screening and fear that non-compliance will lead to criticism. Some 10–30% of women in European screening studies refuse a first invitation and 6–20% of initial attenders refuse further invitations. Some fear associated with screening was expressed by 39% of 125 women in Edinburgh who were interviewed following failure to attend [22]. Among those who do attend, a minority find screening stressful, but say that the feeling of well-being when informed that the breasts are normal adequately compensates for anxiety beforehand.

Some 5–10% of women are recalled after screening as a result of suspicious findings at screening and this may trigger psychiatric illness. An attempt has been made to measure the prevalence and persistence of psychological morbidity following recall in Guildford, a screening centre within the UK (R. Ellman, submitted for publication). The prevalence of psychological morbidity among 300 recalled women was compared with that of 300 women who were screened and found normal. The General Health Questionnaire was filled in by these women at clinics and after an interval of three months. Among the recalled group, distress was slightly more frequent than among the routinely screened group when they were first tested (30% *vs* 25%), but there was no indication of any lasting psychological morbidity among those who did not have cancer: 19% in both groups scored above the standard test threshold at three months.

These reassuring results are probably due to the fact that the recalled women were reviewed by the screening trial staff within less than a week of receiving an appointment and care was taken to explain the reason for recall and give decisive reassurance to those not recommended for biopsy. It was clear from interviews with the women that they rated the communication at the screening and assessment clinic to be of considerably higher quality than that generally experienced with medical services. Prolonged uncertainty about screening results and poor or contradictory explanations may increase the psychological costs of screening and lead to loss of confidence in the screening service.

Psychological Costs of Screening for Cancer Patients

Even when treatments for early and later stage cancers differ little, the psychological costs should be lower when the patient believes she has a better-than-average prognosis. However, among cancer cases detected by screening and included in the Guildford study, the prevalence of psychological morbidity (9/18 had high scores three months after diagnosis) was as high as among breast cancer patients who presented with symptoms. It has been suggested that absence of symptoms may make adjustment to the diagnosis more difficult but no doubts about the necessity of treatment were voiced by any of these women. Despite early diagnosis the women may have been unduly pessimistic: in one case an unrealistic expectation of premature death – 'I looked at the pond and thought this is the last time I shall see it frozen over' – was clearly responsible for unnecessary suffering. An experienced counsellor, by discovering and dispelling misconceptions, can help reduce the psychological distress of cancer patients.

Distress at diagnosis may take the form of anger that screening did not pick up cancer at a stage when cure could be guaranteed. Though staff know the limitations of screening, the anger of such patients may be deeply upsetting. To avoid missing cases, especially if litigation threatens, doctors may too readily recommend biopsy [23]. A clear policy, moral support for staff and a responsible code of medico-legal practice are important in keeping screening costs low.

Earlier diagnosis implies that the consequences of cancer labelling as well as any side-effects of cancer treatment are experienced from an earlier age. For the patient whose life is extended, this is a reasonable cost provided the quality of life after the initial year of adjustment is good, but not so for the patients in whom screening fails to delay metastatic disease. The extreme case of disadvantage is that of a woman who, but for screening, would have remained unaware of having breast cancer throughout her life-time, yet paradoxically, she may express herself as most grateful for screening.

Conclusion

The value of a year of life saved by a screening programme is difficult to assess except by considering analogous situations. The 5-yearly cervical smear screening programme is the only established mass screening programme for cancer in Britain and the cost per year of life saved is probably similar to that for 3-yearly breast cancer screening. Yet the situations are dissimilar: 85% of cervical cancers can be picked up by screening at a pre-invasive stage when cure is almost guaranteed, whereas most breast cancers are invasive by the time they can be detected at screening and have only a guardedly optimistic prognosis. It is the fact that breast cancer is responsible for six times as many deaths as cervical cancer that makes mammographic screening, despite its relatively poor performance, justifiable.

Demand for more frequent screening for breast cancer will grow even with realisation of its shortcomings, but the lesson has been learnt from cervical cancer screening that an equitable distribution of screening resources provides the greatest benefit. Excess demand should be rationed and paid for by the individual, rather than be permitted to cause diversion of public resources from services of greater health benefit.

Information about the costs and the true benefits of breast cancer screening is gradually accumulating and will help determine an optimal level of screening provision but, however precise the information, dispute will continue over the appropriate exchange rates for financial *versus* human value, present *versus* future gain, minor physical or mental distress *versus* premature death and natural *versus* iatrogenic disease.

References

1. Shapiro, S.(1977). Evidence on screening for breast cancer from a randomised trial. *Cancer*, **39**, 2772–2782.
2. Tabar, L., Fagerberg, C.J.G., Gad, A. *et al.* (1985). Reduction in mortality from breast cancer after mass screening with mammography. *Lancet*, **i**, 829–832.
3. Collette, H.J.A., Day, N.E., Rombach, J.J., de Waard, F. (1984). Evaluation of screening for breast cancer in a non-randomised study (the DOM Project) by means of a case-control study. *Lancet*, **i**, 1224–1226.

4. Verbeek, A.L.M., Hendricks, J.H.C.L. *et al.* (1984). Reduction in breast cancer mortality through mass screening with modern mammography. (First results of the Nijmegan Project, 1975–81). *Lancet*, **i**, 1222–1224.
5. Palli, D., Roselli del Turco, M. *et al.* (1986). A case-control study of the efficacy of a non-randomised breast cancer screening program in Florence (Italy). *Int. J. Cancer*, **38**, 501–504.
6. Day, N.E., Chamberlain, J. (1988). Screening for breast cancer: Workshop Report. *Eur. J. Cancer Oncol.*, **24**, 55–59.
7. Working Group, Chariman: Forrest, P. (1987). *Breast Cancer Screening. Report to the Health Ministers of England, Wales, Scotland and Northern Ireland*, HMSO, London.
8. Tabar, L., Fagerberg, G., Day, N.E., Holmberg, L. (1987). What is the optimum interval between mammographic screening examinations? *Brit. J. Cancer*, **55**, 547–551.
9. Bailar, J. (1988). Mammography before 50 years? *J. Amer. Med. Ass.*, **259**, 1548–1549.
10. US Preventive Services Task Force (1987). Recommendations for breast cancer screening. *J. Amer. Med. Ass.*, **257**, 2196.
11. Miller, A.B., Howe, G.R., Wall, C. (1981). The national study of breast cancer screening: protocol for a Canadian randomized controlled trial of screening for breast cancer in women. *Clin. Invest. Med.*, **4**, 227–258.
12. Mant, D., Vessey, M.P., Neil, A., McPherson K., Jones, L. (1987). Breast self-examination and breast cancer stage at diagnosis. *Brit. J. Cancer*, **55**, 207–211.
13. Baines, C.J. (1983). Some thoughts on why women don't do breast self-examination. *Canad. Med. Ass. J.*, **128**, 255–256.
14. Sickles, E.A., Filly, F.A., Callen, P.W. (1983). Breast cancer detection with ultrasonography and mammography: comparison using state-of-the-art equipment. *AJR*, **140**, 843–845.
15. Gravelle, H.S.E., Simpson, P.R., Chamberlain, J. (1982). Breast cancer screening and health service costs. *J. Hlth. Econ.*, **1**, 185–207.
16. Laara, E., Day, N.E., Hakama, M. (1987). Trends in mortality from cervical cancer in the Nordic countries: association with organised screening programmes. *Lancet*, **i**, 1247–1249.
17. Alexander, F.E., Roberts, M.M., Huggins, A., Muir, B. (In press). The use of risk factors to allocate schedules for breast cancer screening. *J. Epidem. Commun. Hltl.*.
18. Feig, S.A. (1984). Benefits and risks of mammography. *Recent Results in Cancer Research*, **90**, 11–27.
19. Moskowitz, M., Garside, P. (1982). Evidence of breast cancer mortality reduction: aggressive screening in women under age 50. *AJR*, **138**, 911–916.
20. Nielsen, M., Thomsen, J., Primdahl, S., Dyreborg, U., Andersen, J. (1987). Breast cancer and atypia among young and middle-aged women: a study of 100 medico-legal autopsies. *Brit. J. Cancer*, **56**, 814–819.
21. Skrabanek, P. (1988). The physician's responsibility to the patient. *Lancet*, **i**, 1155–1156.
22. Maclean, U., Sinfield, D., Klein, S., Harnden, B. (1984). Women who decline breast screening. *J. Epidem. Commun. Hlth.*, **38**, 278–283.
23. Hall, F.M. (1986). Screening mammography – potential problems on the horizon. *New Engl. J. Med.*, **314**, 53–55.

Chapter 10

Prospects for Breast Cancer Prevention

BASIL A. STOLL

Previous chapters have shown that women with an increased susceptibility to breast cancer can be recognised by certain characteristics in their life history which may indicate factors capable of promoting or stimulating breast cancer growth. Measures taken to avoid or counteract these factors in a susceptible woman may arrest progression to frank cancer and lead to dormancy in the growth. This may enable her to live out her natural span of life before the cancer can manifest clinically, and in this sense is equivalent to prevention of the disease.

Until recently, measures proposed for this purpose have involved an attempt either to interfere with oestrogen production in the body or else to counteract the stimulant effect of oestrogen on breast cancer growth. More recently, chemical agents have been recognised which can reverse abnormal cell growth or premalignant changes in breast tissue, and these agents similarly can cause dormancy in cancer growth. The current prospects for breast cancer prevention will be discussed under the following headings;

- Approaches to prevention
- Manipulating ovarian function
- Tamoxifen and other antioestrogenic agents
- Dietary or chemical inhibition of cancer growth
- Prophylactic mastectomy.

Approaches to Prevention

Cancer of the breast in the human is thought to be initiated as a result of irreversible damage to the nucleus of a cell, either by viruses, chemicals in the environment or natural background radioactivity. Such damage is probably common and likely to occur in a high proportion of the population. However, subsequent step-by-step progression towards invasive cancer depends on further stimulation by hormonal or other promoting factors. These factors operate over an interval of 10–15 years between the original initiating damage and the time when frankly invasive cancer becomes manifest clinically.

At present, we are unable either to avoid the initiating damage to cell nuclei or to reverse its changes in the DNA once they have occurred. However, the influence of the subsequent promoting factors is reversible, so that it is possible to extend the latent interval between the first genetic change and the final appearance of cancer. The usual length of this latent interval may be estimated from the report that women aged between 10 and 59 at the time they were exposed to the atomic bomb explosions in 1945, began to show an increased incidence of breast cancer only after the lapse of 14 years [1]. The incidence continued to rise for 30 years after the radiation exposure.

The important role of ovarian hormones in promoting breast cancer in the latent interval is shown by the report that those women who were aged over 50 at the time of the atomic explosion did not show any increased susceptibility to breast cancer [1]. Moreover, girls who were under 10 at the time of the explosion did not begin to show an increased incidence of breast cancer until 21 years later, suggesting that the latent interval was prolonged because of the need for ovarian hormones to appear and promote cancer growth.

There is other epidemiological evidence on the role of ovarian hormones in cancer promotion. Some types of benign breast disease known to predispose to the development of subsequent breast cancer (e.g., fibrocystic disease associated with cysts or tender nodules) are found to be associated with deficient progesterone secretion by the ovary in the years before the onset of the menopause. The peak incidence of fibrocystic disease is 10–15 years before that of breast cancer, and this observation, together with that on the atomic bomb survivors, suggests that an observation period of about 15 years would be necessary to assess the benefit of a clinical trial of hormonal manipulation in the prevention of breast cancer.

In the present state of knowledge, attempts at breast cancer prevention are directed to the latent interval after cancer initiation. It is believed that agents which are able to switch off particular 'growth factors' may maintain a dormant state in the potentially malignant cell, and that examples of such agents are sex hormones or the chemical agents discussed later. However, recent identification in breast cancer or specific oncogenes (variants of normal genes) offers a possibility of using specific antagonists to the abnormal growth factors produced by these genes. For example TGF beta is a growth inhibiting factor which is found to be secreted by some breast cancers and its concentration is known to be decreased by the action of oestrogen [2]. Increasing the level of this growth factor in breast tissue should enable us to inhibit the growth of breast cancer. Alternatively, it may be possible to block the binding sites in the tumour for growth stimulating factors such as epidermal growth factor [3].

Is it possible to select women at high risk for an attempt at prevention? Although clinical criteria of high risk are used at present, susceptible women are likely to be identified in the future through genetic markers. Postulated markers of growth factors which are thought to stimulate breast cancer growth include 52 K protein in cancer cells [4], over-expression of the P21 ras protein in breast tissue [5] and abnormal fibroblasts in the skin [6]. Once we have found genetic markers which are proved to be linked with susceptibility to breast cancer, it would allow monitoring to be focused on specific members of a family group.

Although we can do nothing to avoid the natural background radioactivity which may initiate breast cancer, we should advise against exposure to additional radiation which may accelerate the development of the disease. Thus, women at high risk to breast cancer should avoid unnecessary chest X-rays, particularly before the age of 50. A similar warning applies to overuse of mammography in younger women.

In discussing possible methods of counteracting promoting factors, it needs to be emphasised that these are likely to be different in breast cancer which manifests in premenopausal women from those which apply to postmenopausal women [7]. Thus, for premenopausal Caucasian women, the major clinical risk factors are a family history of the disease in mother or sister, delay before first full-term pregnancy, onset of menstruation at a relatively younger age and incomplete breast feeding of children. For postmenopausal women, on the other hand, the major risk factors are delayed onset of the menopause and the presence of abnormal obesity, although delayed first pregnancy may also be involved. Thus, the implication of a family history of the disease is relatively less important if the breast cancer appears after the menopause.

The term 'secondary prevention' of breast cancer is commonly used in the literature and refers to screening programmes aiming to diagnose a fully developed cancer when it is small in size. Most of the current preventive activity is directed towards such 'secondary prevention' but this is unfortunately too late for many patients. Even if detected by a screening programme when the tumour is too small to be felt, the disease is often found to have spread beyond the primary site.

Manipulating Ovarian Function

The established risk factors discussed in previous chapter suggest that oestrogen, originating either from the ovary, adrenal gland or food intake, is likely to favour the development of breast cancer. Although measurements of circulating oestrogen levels in patients with the disease or their relatives have shown no clear correlation with risk (see Chapter 4), these measurements may not reflect actual levels in breast tissue at critical times in its development. It is postulated that a woman's susceptibility to breast cancer might be decreased by avoiding or counteracting oestrogen environments which favour progression of the disease. Methods which have been suggested include (a) mimicking pregnancy changes in the breasts of teenage girls; (b) prematurely stopping ovarian secretion of oestrogen in middle-aged women; (c) mimicking the effect of delayed onset of menstruation in teenage girls; (d) prolonging breast feeding as long as is practicable.

Mimicking Pregnancy Changes

A full-term pregnancy occurring within five years of the onset of menstrual activity reduces a woman's risk of familial breast cancer by over 50% [8]. It is postulated that full activity in the cells lining the mild ducts may protect against cancer promoters and there is experimental evidence to support the hypothesis. Thus, in rats where breast cancer is easily induced by feeding virgin females with the chemical agent DMBA, the cancer can be prevented by following the chemical induction by pregnancy. It can also be prevented from appearing by administering high dosage of oestradiol, low dosage of oestradiol or a combination of oestrogen and progestogen. All these hormonal methods have in common that they lead to maturation of the secretory cells lining the breast ducts [9]. How practicable are similar procedures in the human?

One suggested method is the administration of low dosage of oestradiol, an oestrogen whose level is increased 1000 fold in the blood during pregnancy [9]. However, such trials would need to be investigated in primates before they can be applied in humans. At that stage, we would still need to define the maximum dose and duration of treatment before we can consider trials of oestradiol in teenage girls with a family history of breast cancer.

Of more immediate practical interest is the induction of a 'pseudopregnancy' as used successfully for treating endometriosis in premenopausal women. Treatment is usually given continuously for 6–12 months, and a typical hormone combination used is ethinyl oestradiol 30 micrograms together with levonorgestrel 250 micrograms. (An identical combination is widely used as an oral contraceptive.) Is it then feasible to protect girls at high risk to breast cancer by giving a suitable combination of oestrogen and progestogen? The difficulty is to decide at which age it should be started and to identify the optimal ratio of the two hormones. We would also need to use the lowest quantity of each agent in order to avoid possible side effects. An ideal combination could act as an oral contraceptive and at the same time protect against breast cancer (see Chapter 8).

Until such 'pseudopregnancy' regimes have been tested it may be justifiable to advise girls belonging to very high risk families to plan for children as early as possible in their childbearing years. The advantage of possibly reducing breast cancer risk might outweigh some of the economic considerations which often lead young couples to postpone their first child.

Premature Menopause

A clear relationship has been noted between susceptibility to breast cancer and a woman's age at the time of either natural or artificially-induced menopause (see Chapter 4). Practically all studies agree that postmenopausal women with breast cancer have gone through the natural menopause at a later average age than have normal women, and that the younger the age of a women at the time of menopause, the lower her risk of developing breast cancer subsequently.

Again, studies have shown a lower frequency of castration (either by removal or irradiation of the ovaries) among breast cancer cases compared to controls. Cessation of menstruation appears to be protective only if ovarian activity is stopped; removal of the uterus without the ovaries does not alter the risk. Again, as for the natural menopause, the degree of protection afforded by stopping ovarian function is inversely related to the age at which it was done. The protective effect of removal of the ovaries is thought to last at least 30 years [10].

Although the practice of hysterectomy is widespread in Western countries, removal of the ovaries at the same time is relatively rare because of the natural desire of most women to delay the manifestations of the menopause for as long as possible. However, in the case of the woman at high risk to breast cancer, it is now recognised that modern hormone replacement therapy (by a combination of low dosage oestrogen together with progestogen) can provide adequate protection against menopausal symptoms yet avoid the danger of endometrial cancer associated with oestrogen-only replacement therapy. For such women, therefore, removal of the ovaries should be performed at the same time as hysterectomy. There is no evidence that hormone replacement therapy by a combination of low-dose oestrogen with added progestogen carries any danger of stimulating breast cancer, and in fact, it may even diminish the risk (see Chapter 8).

Delaying Onset of Menstruation

The onset of menstruation at a relatively early age increases a woman's risk of breast cancer and this may be a factor in the high incidence of the disease among Western women where menstruation tends to begin much earlier than it used to. Ovarian activity is triggered off by the pituitary gland and this in turn is triggered by a controlling centre in the hypothalamus. It is postulated that girls manifest puberty when they achieve a set body fat content, and because of better nutrition in modern society, it is now being reached at an earlier age.

It is reported that women who were former athletes have a significantly lower risk of breast cancer than do non-athletes [11]. Such girls tend to start menstruating at 15, which is 3 years later than average. Obese girls tends to have an earlier onset of puberty than do normal weight girls while female athletes and ballet dancers tend to have a later onset. In the latter groups, strenuous physical exercise may be as important as the lower body fat content because male athletes show similar abnormalities to the females in gonadotrophin secretion. (It is thought that repeated high levels of stress hormones secreted in competitions may cause suppression of gonadotrophin secretion by the pituitary gland.)

Vigorous exercise may therefore be recommended for adolescent girls both to inhibit fat deposits and to inhibit reproductive hormones, and in the presence of a strong family history of breast cancer, this might be an added incentive. It is now possible to delay the onset of menstruation also by treatment with analogues of the hypothalamic hormone LHRH. They could be used to inhibit the secretion of pituitary gonadotrophin for 2 or 3 years, although the long-term effect of such a procedure has not yet been established.

Breast feeding

Recent reports have revived a longstanding hypothesis that prolongation of breast feeding may protect a woman against subsequent development of breast cancer [12, 13]. The longer the total duration of breast feeding the greater the protection, and the benefit seems to be largely confined to breast cancer developing in premenopausal women. It is uncertain whether the advantage of prolonged breast feeding results from its effect in delaying the re-establishment of menstruation after pregnancy (thus decreasing length of exposure to oestrogen), or whether the breast tissue changes associated with prolonged lactation protect the duct lining against subsequent development of cancer.

If its value is proven, it may encourage women at high risk to persist with breast feeding of their infants as long as possible. On the other hand, it may be that the women who is not able to nurse well may have some underlying hormonal imbalance which might also predispose to breast cancer. We need more information as to the *reason* why such women do not persist in feeding.

We noted above that a major factor decreasing the risk of breast cancer in premenopausal women is a full-term pregnancy at a younger age while miscarriages are not protective. (Some reports suggest that an early miscarriage may even increase the risk.) These observations suggest that *early* pregnancy changes in breast tissue are not adequate but only full-term pregnancy with its associated full lactation changes in the secretory epithelium can block the effects of promoting factors for breast cancer.

Tamoxifen and Other Antioestrogenic Mechanisms

The antioestrogen tamoxifen might be effective in delaying the clinical appearance of breast cancer. This agent has been used for about 20 years in the treatment of advanced breast cancer, both postmenopausal and premenopausal. More recently, its administration as adjuvant therapy after primary treatment of early breast cancer has been shown to decrease the rate of relapse and increase the overall survival rate.

These findings have led some groups to advocate its trial as preventive therapy in women considered to be at high risk for developing breast cancer [14, 15]. The criteria used for selecting women for such preventive therapy differs between trials, but include early age at the onset of menstruation, older age at menopause, delayed first full-term pregnancy, family history of breast cancer in mother or sister, history of certain types of benign disease of the breast, abnormal obesity, abnormal mammography pattern and high levels of free oestradiol in the blood.

An advantage of tamoxifen is that it is well tolerated and its short-term side effects are minimal, especially in postmenopausal women. In premenopausal women it often stops menstruation but there is usually a return to normal after stopping administration. Few patients need to have the drug stopped because of intolerance and although a slightly raised risk of thrombosis has been suggested, it is not proven [16]. If the agent is to be given for many years in the hope of decreasing risk of breast cancer, we need to be certain that it does not cause damage to the normal target organs of sex hormones such as bones, ovary, uterus and pituitary gland.

Thus, a trial of tamoxifen as preventive therapy is recommended by one group only for older women (age range 50–70) and for 5 years in the first place [14]. It is not generally recommended for women of childbearing age, but one trial involves women aged 40–49 who give a history of breast cancer in mother or sister [15] and such women are advised to practise contraception while on the drug. Tamoxifen is given either for 3 months or 3 years in this trial, but extrapolation from animal observations suggests that tamoxifen administration for 5–10 years may be necessary to delay the appearance of breast cancer in the human [17].

As a disadvantage of tamoxifen, it has been suggested that patients who may eventually develop breast cancer after attempts to delay it by tamoxifen administration, may show tumours unresponsive to treatment by the agent [18]. This possibility is purely theoretical because patients who have received adjuvant tamoxifen therapy after primary surgery for breast cancer are just as likely to show response to the agent if they relapse as are patients who have not received this antioestrogen [19].

What about other antioestrogenic methods in prevention of breast cancer? It has been shown that oestrogen levels are reduced in premenopausal women who smoke more than 15 cigarettes daily [20] and that in postmenopausal women, the higher oestrogen levels usually associated with increasing body weight are not found in smokers [21]. While smoking (and its associated reduced oestrogen level) is shown to be associated with a reduced risk of endometrial cancer, there is no evidence of a reduced risk of breast cancer.

There is increasing evidence that progestogen may under certain circumstances protect a woman against the cancer-promoting effect of oestrogen (see Chapter 8). The use of a low-dose oestrogen/progestogen combination as hormone replacement therapy may thus protect postmenopausal women against breast cancer if optimal formulation can be established.

Dietary or Chemical Inhibition of Cancer Growth

Reduction of Dietary Fat

In postmenopausal women a major factor contributing to high risk of breast cancer is abnormal obesity and there are several lines of evidence pointing to the importance of dietary factors in the development of breast cancer (see Chapter 6). Reduction of dietary fat has therefore been suggested as a means of decreasing susceptibility to breast cancer, particularly in women with a family history of the disease. Reduction of dietary fat has already been proposed as a means of reducing the frequency of heart disease, strokes and bowel cancers, and it has been suggested that the proportion of the daily calorie intake represented by fat should be reduced from the present 40% to 20%. Such a reduction could be achieved without a major disturbance in dietary habits, but unfortunately, we are still uncertain as to the relative dangers for breast cancer of fat from animal sources as opposed to total fat in the diet.

The National Cancer Institute in the USA has begun two pilot studies to assess possible benefit from lowering fat in the diet of women at risk for breast cancer [22]. The first group are women between the ages of 45 and 69 known to have several high risk factors; the second group are women who have already had one breast removed for cancer and are therefore at risk for cancer of the opposite breast. Fat deposits are thought to be the site of much of the oestrogen production in women after the menopause. We do not known the optimal age at which attempts should be made to reduce obesity, but the years around the menopause when the tendency to obesity increases may be the most suitable.

The importance of dietary factors in susceptibility to breast cancer is difficult to interpret (see Chapter 6). High levels of some aspect of the diet may imply low levels of another, so that a high intakc of meats or fats may be associated with a low intake of vegetable or other food. It has therefore been suggested that even if it were possible to change most women's diet over a period of several decades, an effect on breast cancer risk is unlikely to be observed [23].

Role of Vitamins

Several vitamins and their precursors have been widely investigated in relation to their ability to reduce the risk of breast cancer. They include vitamin A and its precursor beta carotene, vitamin C and its precursor alpha tocopherol, and vitamin D. Although considerable attempts have been made to relate the importance of each vitamin to human susceptibility to breast cancer (see Chapter 6) their relative roles are difficult to disentangle because they tend to be associated with each other in nature.

Epidemiological studies on the role of diet are usually based on national or case control studies and there are conflicting reports as to whether breast cancer is more common in women with a low vitamin A intake [24]. In the case of the individual, there is rarely enough dietary information over a long period of time to enable reliable conclusions to be drawn. Attempts have therefore been made to correlate blood levels of vitamin A or its precursor with the risk of breast cancer, but to date they have been unsuccessful [25].

Retinoids (the family of natural and synthetic analogues of vitamin A) offer the greatest promise as a therapeutic agent. When given to rats immediately after treatment by breast cancer-inducing chemicals, they reduce the incidence and delay the appearance of the tumors. Giving retinoids *in addition* to other tumour-restraining methods (such as removal of the ovaries or the administration of tamoxifen) will reduce the cancer incidence more than does either method by itself. It is not clear whether retinoid inhibition of cancer growth results from counteracting steps in tumour promotion or from subsequent delay in progression from the premalignant stage into frank invasive cancer.

Retinoids can also act on some fully developed cancers and have been shown to suppress the growth of skin, lung and bladder cancers but not, so far, of breast cancer. The major problem in using them for cancer prevention is to find suitable retinoids which are non-toxic at effective dosage. One agent N-(4-hydroxyphenyl) retinamide (HPR) is currently under trial in women who have already had one breast removed and are therefore at risk for cancer of the opposite breast [26].

Vitamin C has been shown to cause regression in premalignant tumours of the rectum, but so far has not been shown active in breast tumours. It is thought to act by blocking oxidative damage to DNA by free radicals. With regard to vitamin D as a possible preventive in human breast cancer, the cells have been shown to carry a receptor for 1,25 dihydroxy vitamin D [27]. Also it is reported that the agent can inhibit proliferation of breast cancer cells [28], possibly by altering calcium levels inside the cell. More information is required from animal studies before clinical application of vitamins to breast cancer prevention can be considered.

Chemical Inhibition

During the past 10–15 years it has been shown in experimental animals that changes leading to cancer may be blocked by synthetic chemical agents. Stages in tumour promotion may be reversed by some, while others may delay the final progression from the premalignant stage into frank invasive cancer. Groups of chemicals which are being investigated include *antioxidant agents* used in food preservation, compounds of *selenium* (a tracer element found both in animals and man) and certain *flavones* and *indoles* found in some vegetables. All have been found to protect experimental animals against chemical induction of cancer.

Antioxidant chemicals have been shown to inhibit cancer development in experimental animals. They act either by detoxicating carcinogenic agents or by blocking damage to DNA by free radicals. The group includes the trace element selenium and vitamin C, apart from chemicals such as butylated hydroxyarisole (BHA) and butylated hydroxytolene (BHT) which are widely used in food preservation. Feeding animals with these latter agents protects them against the enhancing effect of a high-fat diet on chemically-induced breast cancer in rats. They appear to be more effective against saturated fats than against unsaturated fats.

Selenium acts as an essential trace element both in animals and man, and several studies have shown higher cancer mortality in certain populations with low seleniua intake or blood levels (see Chapter 6). Selenium administration has been found to protect animals against the enhancing effect of a high-fat diet on chemically-induced breast cancer and can even reverse precancerous changes. A combination of selenium and retinoids will reduce the incidence of such cancers more than does either agent alone [23]. Their use against human cancer requires more investigation.

Flavones and indoles are found in cruciferous vegetables such as brussels sprouts, cabbage, turnips, broccoli and cauliflower. Some members of these chemical groups have been found effective in inhibiting the growth of chemically-induced breast cancer in animals. However, one survey of breast cancer patients and controls [23] has shown no difference in their intake of cruciferous vegetables or vitamin C, but did show a relatively low intake of vitamin A among postmenopausal breast cancer patients. As noted above, there are considerable problems in assessing the influence of vitamin intake on the development of a disease with multiple promoting factors and a long latent interval such as breast cancer.

Prophylactic Mastectomy

In rare cases, subcutaneous removal of both breasts with reconstruction has been advised in women at the highest risk to cancer and with a marked cancer phobia. This would apply especially to younger women with markedly fibrocystic breasts which are difficult to examine. Surgery might also be considered in women with a history of multiple family members suffering from breast cancer (particularly if they occurred before the menopause), a history of multiple breast biopsies or a high-risk pattern in the mammogram [29] (see Chapter 3).

Sometimes a patient treated for early breast cancer in one breast may be considered for prophylactic removal of the opposite breast, particularly if the opposite breast has shown a precancerous biopsy or has a high-risk pattern in the mammogram. Again, such findings are more worrisome in a patient with a history of premenopausal breast cancer in a mother or sister.

A difficult surgical decision arises in the case of lobular cancer *in situ*. This is a type of non-invasive cancer predominantly affecting premenopausal women and tending to involve both breasts. About one quarter of all cases progress to cancer either in one or both breasts although it may be delayed for 20 years or more [30]. Thus, some authorities advise mastectomy at the time of original diagnosis while some go even further and suggest that both breasts be removed. It would depend on the decision of the patient after full information is provided.

Reconstruction of the breast after primary mastectomy is becoming increasingly popular, and is usually done at the same operation. Subcutaneous mastectomy can be offered to such women because it preserves the skin of the breast and also the nipple. However, as it leaves some breast tissue intact under the skin and nipple, it offers a less sure safeguard than does complete mastectomy. Different types of reconstruction have their advocates. Silicone implants are the most common, involving an envelope containing silicone gel or saline. In order to minimise the scar tissue which forms around it, an envelope can be filled gradually to stretch the tissues more slowly. An alternative type of reconstruction is to use a flap of skin and muscle taken either from the shoulder region (latissimus dorsi flap) or from the abdominal wall (rectus abdominis flap). The plastic surgeon has the duty to explain the limitations and advantages of each method to the patient, and to offer her the choice.

Conclusion

Recognised risk criteria do not fully account for the variation seen between individuals in their susceptibility to breast cancer. Nevertheless, an attempt to avoid or counteract the promoting factors assumed to be associated with risk criteria might prolong the latent interval before the tumour manifests clinically or else delay progression from the precancerous stage. These goals may be achieved by hormonal, dietary or chemical means.

Clinical trials have been set up both in the USA and Europe to assess whether the use of tamoxifen, vitamin A analogues or low-fat diets can delay the appearance of breast cancer in women known to be at high risk to the disease. It will take several years to evaluate these trials. While awaiting the results (or the development of some other methods of prevention), the physician must help each woman to make a personal decision, based on her own personal evaluation of the likelihood of benefit in relation to the anxiety or complications involved in a monitoring or prevention programme. The present choice is essentially between regular screening, bilateral mastectomy, dietary changes, tamoxifen therapy or early termination of ovarian function.

The most hopeful prospect is for an oestrogen-progestogen combination which might be used for family planning in premenopausal women or replacement therapy in postmenopausal women, and at the same time protect against breast cancer.

References

1. Tokunaga, M., Norman, J.E., Asano, M. *et al.* (1979). Malignant breast tumours among atomic bomb survivors. *J. Nat. Cancer Inst.*, **62** 1347–1359.
2. Roberts, A.B., Anzano, M.A., Wakefield, L.M. *et al.* (1985). Type B transforming growth factor. A bifunctional regulator of cellular growth. *Proc. Nat. Acad. Sci.*, **82**, 119–123.
3. Sainsbury, J.R.C., Farndon, J.R., Sherbet, G.V., Harris, A.L. (1985). Epidermal growth factor receptor and oestrogen receptors in human breast cancer. *Lancet*, **i**, 364–366.
4. Garcia, M., Salazar, R.G., Pages, A. *et al.* (1986). Distribution of 52K oestrogen regulated protein in benign breast disease and other tissue by immunohistochemistry. *Cancer Res.*, **46**, 3734–3738.
5. Ohuchi, N., Thor, A., Page, D.L. *et al.* (1986). Expression of 21K ras protein in a spectrum of benign and malignant human mammary tissues. *Cancer Res.*, **46**, 2511–2519.
6. Haggie, J.A., Sellwood, R.A., Howell, A. *et al.* (1987). Fibroblasts from relatives of patients with hereditary breast cancer show fetal-like behaviour *in vitro*. *Lancet*, **i**, 1455–1457.
7. Wynder, E.L., MacCornack, F.A., Stellman, S.D. (1978). Epidemiology of breast cancer in 785 United States Caucasian women. *Cancer*, **41**, 2341–2354.
8. MacMahon, B., Cole, P., Brown, J.B. (1973). Etiology of human breast cancer; a review. *J. Nat. Cancer Inst.*, **50**, 21–42.
9. Lemon, H.M. (1987). Antimammary carcinogenic activity of estriol. *Cancer*, **60**, 2873–2881.
10. Trichopoulos, D., MacMahon, B., Cole, P. (1972). Menopause and breast cancer risk. *J. Nat. Cancer Inst.*, **48**, 605–611.
11. Frisch, R.E., Wyshak, G., Albright, N.L. *et al.* (1985). Lower prevalence of breast cancer among former college athletes. *Brit. J. Cancer*, **52**, 885–891.
12. Byers, T., Graham, S., Rzepka, T. *et al.* (1985). Lactation and breast cancer; evidence for a negative association in premenopausal women. *Amer. J. Epidem.*, **121**, 664–674.
13. McTiernan, A., Thomas, D.B. (1986). Evidence for a protective effect of lactation on risk of breast cancer in young women. *Amer. J. Epidem*, **124**, 353–358.
14. Cuzick, J., Wang, D.Y., Bulbrook, R.D. (1986). The prevention of breast cancer. *Lancet*, **i**, 83–86.
15. Gazet, J.C., (1985). Tamoxifen prophylaxis for women at high risk of breast cancer. *Lancet*, **ii**, 1119.
16. Auger, M.J., Mackie, M.J. (1988). Effects of tamoxifen on blood coagulation. *Cancer*, **61**, 1316–1319.
17. Jordan, V.C. (1988). *Antiestrogens in Cancer Treatment*. In Stoll, B.A. (ed.), *Endocrine Management of Breast Cancer*, vol 2, S. Karger, Basel, 57–64.

18. Wong, W. (1986). Tamoxifen prophylaxis. *Lancet*, **i**, 264.
19. Muss, H.B., Smith, L.R., Cooper, M.R. (1987). Tamoxifen rechallenge; response to tamoxifen following relapse. *J. Clin. Oncol.*, **5**, 1556–1558.
20. Michnovicz, J.J., Hershcopf, R.J., Naganuna, H. *et al.* (1986). Increased 2-hydroxylation of estradiol as a possible mechanism for the antiestrogenic effect of cigarette smoking. *N. Engl. J. Med.*, **315**, 1305–1309.
21. Lawrence, C., Tessaro, J., Durgerian, S. *et al.* (1987). Smoking, body weight and early stage endometrial cancer. *Cancer*, **59**, 1665–1669.
22. Thomas, D.B., Chu, J. (1986). Nutritional and endocrine factors in reproductive organ cancers. *J. Chron. Dis.*, **39**, 1031–1050.
23. Mettlin, C. (1984). Diet and epidemiology of human breast cancer. *Cancer*, **53**, 605–611.
24. Katsouyanni, K., Willett, W., Trichopoulos, D. *et al.* (1988). Risk of breast cancer among Greek women in relation to nutrient intake. *Cancer*, **61**, 181–185.
25. Marubini, E., Decarli, A., Costa, A. *et al.* (1988). The relationship of dietary intake and serum levels of retinol and beta carotene with breat cancer. *Cancer*, **61**, 173–180.
26. Costa, A., Veronesi, U., Marubini, E. *et al.* (1987). Prevention of contralateral breast cancer with Fenretinide (personal communication).
27. Eisman, J.A., Martin, T.J., MacIntyre, I., Moseley, J.M. (1979). 1,25-Dihydroxy-vitamin D receptor in breast cancer cells. *Lancet*, **ii**, 1335–1336.
28. Frampton, R.J., Ormond, S.A., Eisman, J.A. (1983). Inhibition of human cancer cell growth by 1,25-dihydroxyvitamin D. *Cancer Res.*, **43**, 4443–4447.
29. McKenna, R.J. (1983). Applied cancer prevention in practice. *Cancer*, **51**, 2430–2439.
30. Wolmark, N. (1983). Minimal breast cancer: a major therapeutic dilemma. In Margolese, R.G. (ed.), *Breast Cancer*, Churchill Livingstone, New York, 123–150.

Chapter 11

Counselling Women at High Risk

JOERN BECKMANN

The prospect of contracting breast cancer is frightening for most women. Due to the high frequency of the disease, most women have friends, acquaintances or even family members suffering from it. The unpredictable nature of the disease and the impact of possible surgery make many women live with a hidden fear of contracting breast cancer.

Anxiety Reactions to a Breast Lump

When medical or self-examination shows the presence of a breast lump, a woman's first thought will be: 'It is most probably breast cancer'. Thus, although the vast majority of breast lumps are benign, the finding of a lump combined with the anticipation of breast cancer may provoke a state of near-shock. The resulting pervasive anxiety may give rise to various types of reaction in a woman.

In some cases, a woman will deny her fears, hoping that the tumour will disappear overnight and she may consequently delay seeing a doctor. She may be so paralysed with fear of breast cancer that she may even refuse to face the results of medical examination. In both cases the woman runs the risk of reducing the range of possible treatment available. A more frequent reaction to finding the breast lump is that she is so certain of breast cancer that in her mind she starts preparing herself for death and tries to imagine how her family will carry on without her.

But in every woman, the period between discovering a lump and obtaining the final diagnosis is an extremely stressful time, and at this stage, it is vital for the woman to have the chance of expressing herself to a person whom she can trust. The simple act of being able to put her ideas into words is a great relief for her.

Support by the person she confides in is of great importance to her. The woman is no longer alone, there is someone to help her bear her fears. The person with whom the woman chooses to share her worries must offer her comfort and encouragement but this should not be too exaggerated, otherwise it may block the mental processing of fear and anxiety. It is important to encourage the woman to express herself as much as possible.

Similar support is also the concern of the doctor when he has to tell the patient that the tumour is cancerous and necessitates surgery to the breast. At this stage it is of crucial importance that the doctor is able to explain the diagnosis and its further consequences in an honest and understanding way.

This chapter will deal with psychosocial aspects of breast self-examination, screening for detection of breast cancer, patient delay and optimal information.

Breast Self-examination

On the basis of the scanty information so far available, it is possible to identify a number of psychological and behavioural characteristics in the woman who shows the highest degree of motivation and acceptance of breast self-examination.

1. She is convinced that breast cancer is the worst conceivable disease to develop [1, 2].
2. She engages persistently (particularly if she is under 35) in other preventive health examinations [3].
3. She does not hesitate to consult a doctor when she detects something abnormal in her breast [4].
4. She is quicker to ask for medical examinations than the woman who does not practise breast self-examination. The woman who consults a doctor early is characterized by a combination of anxiety and optimism whereas the woman who fails to see a doctor is dominated by anxiety and pessimism [5].
5. She feels that she is good at performing breast self-examination [6].
6. She is more optimistic about the chances of being cured [1, 5].
7. She is better educated than the non-accepting woman [7].

Mass Screening

The psychological characteristics of women who most consistently participate in breast screening are in many ways similar to those mentioned above for women engaging in breast self-examination. In addition, they lie in the highest income brackets and have relative high job status [8, 9]. Women refusing to participate in breast screening generally see the screening procedure as involving a risk, and they are afraid their lives will be ruined if the screening reveals breast cancer. They are often also of the opinion that one should not create more problems for oneself than those already existing [10].

The factors motivating women to participate in mass screening are identified in a Finnish study as follows: friends 44%, newspapers 29%, television 12%, general practitioners 8%, Society for the Prevention of Cancer 6%, meetings 5%, radio 4%, church 1%, fosters 1%, others 11% [11]. For most women, suspected breast cancer implies a direct and concrete threat to life, body experience, sex identity, sexuality and partner relations in general. While it is natural for a woman to react with anxiety to the prospect of breast cancer, the danger lies in the way this anxiety is handled and the behaviour it induces.

If mechanisms of denial force the woman to dismiss the problem and take up a self-deluding attitude, there is a risk that the women will delay consulting a doctor or, alternatively, may refuse to participate in mass screening for early detection of breast cancer. It is therefore essential that she is offered the positive expectation that the sooner she is examined the better her chances of a successful treatment; and also the more consistently she participates in repetitive screenings, the greater her chances of a favourable prognosis.

Invitations to mass screenings should therefore make use of the woman's anxiety *to motivate her in a positive way*. The motivation should be based on the communication of information about the disease which sill stress the optimistic rather than the frightening elements. This attitude is expressed in the slogan of the Society for the Prevention of Cancer: 'Cancer detected in time is curable'.

There are, of course, possible negative consequences of mass screening for breast cancer, particularly the anxiety-inducing factors. These not only result in unnecessary fears in a large part of the population, but also mean that the woman found to be positive has to live with the diagnosis of cancer of the breast some years sooner than she would otherwise have done (see Chapter 9). The negative psychological consequences of this cannot be ignored.

Statistically, one out of every 14 women develops breast cancer, but is it reasonable that the other 13 must live with an increased awareness of this threatening sword of Damocles of breast cancer? Is it fair that 13 out of 14 women are subject to screening for the purpose of detecting breast cancer in the fourteenth woman some years sooner? From a medical point of view the answer to such questions must be 'yes' if breast cancer is to be identified as early as possible in order to improve the prospects of successful therapy. But what is the consumer's opinion? What is the attitude of all the women who are subjected to a mass invitation to breast screening? These factors have not been examined adequately.

There is another possible risk: that the constant fear of mutilation and death from the development of breast cancer may impair the resistance of some vulnerable women. This might render them more susceptible to the disease, or else increase the mortality of those already attacked by the disease. The existence of such a risk is underlined by two reports [12, 13] that breast cancer patients showing a fighting spirit, optimism and adequate coping mechanisms manifested a significantly lower mortality rate than did women characterized by defeatism, depressive tendencies and helplessness. Further support for the hypothesis may be the finding that an exceptionally high mortality rate due to breast cancer has been found in the black community of Harlem, New York, where monthly breast self-examination, is more frequent among black than among white women [14, 15].

Patient Delay

The term 'delay' refers to the period between symptom detection by the patient and the time when medical attention is sought [16]. Several factors, such as stage of disease, tumour histology, physician or diagnostic delay, knowledge of breast cancer symptoms, patient age, and socio-economic status, have been inconclusively associated with patient delay. This discussion will focus only on the personality characteristics, health behaviour practices or life-styles of women who delay in seeking advice for a symptom suggestive of breast cancer.

The personalities of delayers and non-delayers have been compared in order to determine if psychological factors contribute to the way in which women seek medical care once a breast cancer symptom is self-detected. As a generalisation, those with metastases already present are more likely to be depressed, while patients free of metastases are more anxious and more promptly seek treatment [17, 18].

There is a hypothesis that women who experience pleasurable tactile sensations from their breasts may be less likely to delay seeking medical attention. Though no statistical analysis has been offered to support this, it has been found that fear, anxiety, lack of pleasure in the breast being touched, indecisiveness, negativism, compulsion and guilt feelings are more prevalent among delayers [19]. Another hypothesis suggests that the more precise an individual's body boundary is, the greater is the likely delay. It has been suggested that 'high barrier' patients are more autonomous, feel more secure and less disturbed by breast symptoms, all of which predispose to delaying medical care [20].

A connection between personality, social milieu and a tendency to postpone treatment for breast abnormalities has been investigated, and the results showed that delay depends on life-style and limited knowledge or experience of the medical world [21]. Since fear of mastectomy is related to delaying behaviour in women it is not surprising that a positive biopsy is associated with longer delay. Delayers are also more likely to be postmenopausal and habitual 'deniers'. The health care system may also contribute to length of delay in that not all women have equal access to immediate medical examination [22].

Analysis of 39 psychological factors showed that delay was positively related to avoidance defence. Delayers were also more depressed at the time of their interview in the breast clinic, and they showed more helplessness and a diffuse thinking pattern. A comparison between delayers and non-delayers (defining delay as more than eight weeks) showed that delayers have more inner tension and more inhibition than nondelayers [23]. A study exploring 'intended' delay for breast symptoms showed that the more the interviewee anticipated that her family and friends would recommend monitoring a breast symptom, the more delay was noted. It also showed that the habit of seeking immediate health care after noticing any physical symptom was associated with less delay [24].

It is suggested that a potential breast cancer patient goes through three stages of thinking in the delay process: (1) The woman appraises the actual sensory data (e.g., pain) that causes her to notice symptoms and decides whether there is anything wrong; (2) once an affirmative conclusion is reached, the woman decides whether professional care is needed; (3) if professional care is decided upon, the woman then weighs the cost of care against her barriers to the health system. Furthermore, each decision process is overlaid with coping responses (e.g, home remedies) and emotional response (e.g., fear) along with imagined consequences of the perceived symptoms (e.g, mastectomy) [25].

Optimal Information

In recent years it has been emphasized that every patient should have the right to responsibility for and control of his or her own life. This presupposes optimal information from all professional health-caring groups who must accept that they, as Kierkegaard says 'are not masters but servants, whose most distinguished duty is, through humility, understanding, and love, to discover and understand where their patient is heading, hold her hand and allow themselves to be led'.

Optimal information means telling the patient exactly what she is prepared to receive. Suppression of information about the disease and its development will have the effect of not providing the patient with sufficient information on which to make decisions, thereby not allowing her to take responsibility for her own life. In this process, the therapist must be able to surrender a portion of his power and strength for the benefit of the patient. But optimal information does *not* mean telling the patient everything. Demands are made on the therapist's sensitivity, psychological understanding and ethical attitudes, in order to provide the patient with the amount of information she is ready to receive, at the appropriate point in time.

Optimal information is a process in which the therapist, in a situation of trust and empathy, develops the patient's self-understanding and generates in her the courage to live or die. The physician's fear of telling his patients 'the truth. is often tied to his own still unresolved fear of dying. In other words, the physician often talks to and treats himself. He alleviates pain because it hurts him, and he minimizes his patient's death because he is afraid of his own death. Our understanding of other people includes both conscious and unconscious ways of grasping their meaning. The more we are able to weaken our prejudices, the more we remain open and receptive to what may be taking place inside the other person, the greater is our chance of encountering her as a 'whole human being'.

The concept of truth is of extreme importance in all relationships between people. Not telling the truth means losing one's trustworthiness, and not being trusted means losing one's power and self-respect. But the truth is not always something absolute and objective. It is problematic, especially in a relationship between doctor and patient. A distinction can be made between 'medical truth' and 'patient's truth'. Reaching an identity between medical truth and patient's truth is a permanent challenge to the doctor or the helper, and normally cannot be done immediately, but needs a process of time. It is the doctor's obligation to tell his patient the truth she needs and is prepared to receive is the truth that will help her. Telling her too little or too much is equivalent to violence.

The ultimate ethical demand was made by Kierkegaard in 1859:

> If you really want to help somebody, first of all you must find him where he is and start there. This is the secret of caring. If you cannot do that, it is only an illusion, if you think you can help another human being. Helping somebody implies your understanding more than he does, but first of all you must understand what he understands. If you cannot do that, your understanding will be of no avail. All true caring starts with humiliation. The helper must be humble in his attitude towards the person he wants to help. He must understand that helping is not dominating, but serving. Caring implies patience as well as acceptance of not being right and of not understanding what the other person understands.

References

1. Hobbs, P., Haran, D.W., Pendelton, L.L. (1981). Breast screening by breast self-examination: an evaluation of teaching methods and materials. *Cancer Detect. Prevent.*, **4**, 545–551.

2. Haran, D., Hobbs, P., Pendleton, L.L. (1979). An evaluation of the teaching of breast self-examination for the early detection of breast cancer: factors that affect current awareness and anxiety. In Osborne, D.J., Gruneberg, M.M., Eiser, J.R. (eds.), *Research in Psychology and Medicine: International Conference on Psychology and Medicine, Proceedings*.
3. Turnbull, E.M. (1978). Effect of basic preventive health practices and mass media on the practice of breast self-examination. *Nurs. Res.*, **27**, 98–102.
4. Nichols, S., Waters, W.E. (1983). The practice and teaching of breast self-examination in Southampton. *Publ. Hlth.*, **97**, 816.
5. Sugar, M., Watkins, C. (1961). Some observations about patients with breast mass. *Cancer*, **14**, 979–988.
6. Smith, E.M., Francis, A.M., Polissar, L. (1980). The effect of breast self-examination practices and physician examinations on extent of disease at diagnosis. *Prevent. Med.*, **9**, 409–417.
7. Huguley, C.M., Brown, F.L. (1981). The value of breast self-examination. *Cancer*, **47**, 989–995.
8. Fink, R., Shapiro, E., Roester, R. (1972). Impact of efforts to increase participation in repetitive screenings for early breast cancer detection. *Amer. J. Publ. Hlth.*, **62**, 328–336.
9. Hobbs, P., Smith, A., George, D.W., Wellwood, F.A. (1980). Acceptors and rejectors of an invitation to undergo breast screening compared with those who referred themselves. *J. Epidem. Commun. Hlth.*, **34**, 19–22.
10. French, K., Porter, A.M.D., Robinson, S.E., McCallum, F.M., Howie, J.G.R., Roberts, M.M. (1982). Attendance at a breast screening clinic: a problem of administration or attitudes. *Brit. Med. J.*, **285**, 617–620.
11. Baker, L.H. (1982). Breast cancer detection demonstration project: five-years summary report. *CA (Cancer J. Clinicians)*, **32**, 194–225.
12. Greer, S., Morris, T., Pettingdale, K.W. (1979). Psychological responses to breast cancer: effect and outcome. *Lancet*, **ii**, 785–787.
13. Derogatis, L.R., Abeloff, M.D., Melisaratos, N. (1979). Psychological coping mechanisms and survival time in metastatic breast cancer. *J. Amer. Med. Ass.*, **242**, 504– = 508.
14. Adams, M., Kerner, J.F. (1982). Evaluation of promotional strategies to solve the problem of underutilization of a breast examination/education center in a New York City black community. In: Mettlin, xx. Curtis, xx and Murphy, G.B. (eds.), *Issues in Cancer Screening and Communications: Proceedings*, 151–161.
15. Reeder, S., Berkanowic, E., Marcus, A.C. (1980). Breast cancer detection behaviour among urban women *Publ. Hlth. Rep.*, **95**, 276–281.
16. Antonovsky, A., Hartman, H. (1974). Delay in the detection of cancer: a review of the literature. *Hlth. Educ. Monographs*, 98–128.
17. Green, L.W., Roberts, B.J. (1974). The research literature on why women delay in seeking medical care for breast symptoms. *Hlth. Educ. Monographs*, 129–177.
18. Sugar, M., Watkins, C. (1961). Some observations about patients with a breast mass. *Cancer*, **14**, 979–988.
19. Gold, M.A. (1964). Causes of patient delay in diseases of the breast. *Cancer*, **17**, 564–577.
20. Hammersclag, C.A., Fisher, S., Decosse, J., Kaplan, E. (1964). Breast symptoms and patient delay: psychological variables involved. *Cancer*, **17**, 1480–1485.
21. Cameron, A., Hinton, J. (1968). Delay in seeking treatment for mammary tumours. *Cancer*, **21**, 1121–1126.
22. Greer, S. (1974). Psychological aspects: delay in the treatment of breast cancer. *Proc. Roy. Soc. Med.*, **67**, 470–473.
23. Magarey, C.J., Todd, P.E., Blizzard, F.J. (1975). Measurement of women's attitudes to breast cancer. *Austral. New Zeal. J. Surg.*, **45**, 112.
24. Lutgemeier, I., Rossler, J., Lutgemeier, J., Horst, M. (1979). Verscleppungszeit beim Mammakarzinom und Persoenlichkeitsstruktur. *Onkologie*, **2**, (4), 152–155.

25. Safer, M.A., Tharps, Q.J., Jackson, T.C., Leventhal, H. (1979). Determinants of three stages of delay in seeking care at a medical clinic. *Medical Care*, **17(1)**, 11–29.

Index